"This book does modern medicine a great service by beginning to fill the enormous chasm of missing literature on low back pain. The skilled authors emphasize its cause and illustrate effective treatments. The book is organized with eloquent headings and presented effectively for the primary reader, the patient."

> —David G. Simons, MD, associate voluntary professor at Emory University and coauthor, with Janet Travell, of *Myofascial Pain and Dysfunction: The Trigger Point Manual*, V.1 and V.2

"Sharon Sauer and Mary Biancalana have written a marvelous book that takes the reader from low back pain symptoms to self-management. They have given us a gold mine of information in a user-friendly format. The workbook includes detailed illustrations that are wonderful guides to treatment. Their work is based on the time-tested insights of Janet Travell and David Simons, whose wisdom graces the pages of this fine manual. I can recommend this book to all who suffer from occasional or chronic low back pain."

> —Robert D. Gerwin, MD, associate professor of neurology at Johns Hopkins University in Baltimore, MD

"Sharon Sauer and Mary Biancalana have put together a well-organized and highly practical manual that should be of great use to practitioners of both Western and Eastern medicine. Allopathic and Western-based schools of bodywork training would be notably enriched by the principles and techniques they share. Acupuncturists and Eastern-based bodyworkers will also find new understanding and novel techniques to enhance practice. This material is highly relevant to all who are engaged in the work of relieving pain, and no differential diagnosis of a pain syndrome would be complete without considering myofascial dysfunction. I look forward to using the manual to enhance the care I am able to provide my patients, and hope others will do the same."

> —David W. Miller, MD, FAAP, L.Ac., Dipl. OM, physician at East-West Integrated Medicine, LLC, in Chicago, IL

"*Trigger Point Therapy for Low Back Pain* is essential reading for anyone suffering from low back pain. It gives the best brief explanation of nutrition and pain that I have seen. I recommend this book to anyone with low back pain and to all health care professionals who have patients with low back pain."

> —Tim Taylor, MD, physician at the Pain Relief Home medical practice in Richmond, VA

"This book addresses one of the most common yet frequently ignored causes of chronic low back and pelvic pain—myofascial pain due to trigger points. Sharon Sauer and Mary Biancalana have written a useful book that can help patients identify and treat these pain generators. It contains easy-to-understand drawings and graduated exercises to help prevent recurrence of symptoms, and gives patients some control over their quality of life."

> —Devin J. Starlanyl, coauthor of *Fibromyalgia and Chronic Myofascial Pain*

"A comprehensive and easy-to-understand formula for reducing lower back pain. Special tips are interlaced throughout the book that will help patients and experts effectively reduce and eliminate pain. It is easy to follow and understand, and is packed with information that will help you reclaim your health."

> —Hal Blatman, MD, past president of the American Holistic Medical Association and medical director of Blatman Pain Clinic in Cincinnati, OH

"This book is for everyone from the layperson with low back pain to the medical practitioner who wants to learn effective treatments for myofascial pain. The authors have covered all the essentials: understanding pain that comes from trigger points, examining yourself or your patients, and developing a treatment plan. This book features clear illustrations with descriptions of pain patterns, self-care, exercises and professional techniques that really work. This is a must for everyone who experiences low back pain or treats it professionally!"

> —Angelique C. Mizera, DO, Swedish Covenant Pain Center in Chicago, IL

"Having personally witnessed the results of the authors' work with my chiropractic patients, I can say without hesitation that the method of trigger point therapy demonstrated in this book is a critical component of a successful back pain relief and spinal health program. All my patients and staff members will be getting a copy."

> —Justin Tossing, DC, physical medicine and rehabilitation specialist

"The good news is that back pain is usually treatable. Unfortunately, most physicians are simply not trained to treat pain without drugs or surgery. Got back pain? This book can help you get pain-free—now!"

> —Jacob Teitelbaum, MD, medical director of the national Fibromyalgia and Fatigue Centers

Trigger Point Therapy for Low Back Pain

A SELF-TREATMENT WORKBOOK

Sharon Sauer, CMTPT, LMT
Mary Biancalana, MS, CMTPT, LMT

New Harbinger Publications, Inc.

Publisher's Note

This publication is designed to provide accurate and authoritative information in regard to the subject matter covered. It is sold with the understanding that the publisher is not engaged in rendering medical, psychological, financial, legal, or other professional services. If expert assistance or counseling is needed, the services of a professional should be sought. All readers experiencing pain of any kind should first consult a physician to rule out nonmyofascial origins of pain.

Care has been taken to confirm the accuracy of the information presented and to describe generally accepted practices. However, the authors, editors, and publisher are not responsible for errors or omissions or for any consequences from application of the information in this book and make no warranty, express or implied, with respect to the contents of the publication.

Some medical devices presented in this publication may have Food and Drug Administration (FDA) clearance for limited use in restricted research settings. It is the responsibility of the health care provider to ascertain the FDA status of each drug or device planned for use in their clinical practice.

Cover image as well as figures 5.1-5.2, 6.1-6.7, 7.1-7.3, 8.1-8.3, 9.1-9.2, 10.1-10.4, 11.1-11-2, 13.1-13.2, 14.1-14.2, abd 17.1-17.2 were previously published in Travell and Simons' *Myofascial Pain and Dysfunction: The Trigger Point Manual*, Second Edition. 1999. Lippincott, WIlliams, and Wilkins: Baltimore MD, and are reproduced with permission of the copyright holder.

Figures 5.21, 6.43-6.44, 7.28, 8.29, 12.64-12.67, and 13.19 are used with permission from the Gebauer Company.

Distributed in Canada by Raincoast Books

Copyright © 2010 by Sharon Sauer and Mary Biancalana
New Harbinger Publications, Inc.
5674 Shattuck Avenue
Oakland, CA 94609
www.newharbinger.com

FSC
Mixed Sources
Product group from well-managed
forests and other controlled sources

Cert no. SW-COC-002283
www.fsc.org
© 1996 Forest Stewardship Council

Cover design by Amy Shoup; Text design by Michele Waters-Kermes; Acquired by Jess O'Brien; Edited by Jasmine Star

Printed in the United States of America

Library of Congress Cataloging-in-Publication Data

Sauer, Sharon.
  Trigger point therapy for low back pain : a self-treatment workbook / Sharon Sauer and Mary Biancalana ; foreword by Bernard E. Filner.
    p. cm.
  Includes bibliographical references and index.
  ISBN 978-1-57224-563-1
  1. Backache--Popular works. 2. Myofascial pain syndromes--Popular works. I. Biancalana, Mary. II. Title.
  RD771.B217T75 2010
  617.5'64--dc22
                                2010002417

12   11   10

10   9   8   7   6   5   4   3   2   1   First printing

Contents

Foreword

Pain is the most common symptom for which people seek medical treatment. Nonmalignant soft-tissue pain probably accounts for the vast majority of these visits. Myofascial pain, or soft tissue pain, is the most common type of pain. And the low back, the particular focus of this book, is the area most commonly affected. These facts alone make this an important text. In addition, the approach taken by Sharon and Mary makes it a unique contribution to the field.

The first few chapters of this book provide a clear explanation of myofascial pain syndromes, their signs and symptoms (signs being objective findings, and symptoms being subjective complaints). The explanation of referred pain is of particular importance in understanding and treating this common but frequently overlooked condition. Detailed self-treatment techniques are introduced to help people along the path to recovery.

The muscle chapters and symptom index associate specific symptoms and signs with specific muscles, encouraging people to investigate and understand their condition and then begin to treat it. This knowledge and the hope it engenders will begin the process of decreasing the suffering that goes along with chronic pain. Don't underestimate the impact of regaining a measure of control over this part of your life.

The last two chapters cover topics applicable to all the muscles discussed in this book: range of motion exercises and general perpetuating factors involved in low back pain.

The authors clearly expect readers to rely on their personal physician as the primary resource in evaluating their pain. Once nonmyofascial causes have been considered and ruled out, it makes sense to focus on myofascial pain and dysfunction as the primary problem. For many people, the assistance of a well-trained practitioner may be essential. To that end, each chapter contains a section aimed at practitioners who aren't widely acquainted with or highly skilled at treating myofascial syndromes. This grassroots approach to helping health care providers become more knowledgeable and skilled has the potential to rapidly increase access to skilled myofascial treatment for many common conditions involved in chronic pain.

I've personally seen countless cases in which myofascial pain turned out to be the decisive element in chronic pain syndromes such as migraine, nerve entrapment, neuropathic pain, arthritis, and disk herniation. And time after time, when the myofascial pain was treated, the chronic syndrome was either eliminated or greatly eased in frequency and severity of symptoms.

The question remains: Will the growing demand for treatment increase the availability of these services? Certain factors are aligned against adequate and timely treatment of chronic pain in this country, including lack of training (in and after medical school and in continuing education opportunities) and the resulting limited number of well-trained providers. This book aims at combating the problem from the bottom up. The greatest impediments to the approach described here come from insurance carriers (private and governmental) that often don't or won't cover this helpful therapy.

It's strange that the staggering cost of surgery and drug therapy for chronic back pain and the additional costs of worker's compensation and disability don't drive either the insurance carriers or the government to evaluate more carefully the low-cost alternatives that so often work. It's clear that inadequate reimbursement (or no reimbursement) discourages practitioners from entering this field, and threatens the continued availability of services from those already in the field. Doctors and therapists often can't provide these services and still maintain the financial viability of their practice. This last problem is likely to be solved only through the political process of health care reform, and given the power of existing big players in the medical system, that seems like a very long shot indeed, at least at this point in time.

In my seventeen years of practice as an anesthesiologist and twenty years of treating chronic soft-tissue pain (the first ten mentored by Dr. Janet Travell), these problems have not been solved from the top down. I've come to the conclusion that the primary premise of this book is the right approach now. It is my hope and expectation that this book will be a turning point in the movement to raise the quality and availability of chronic pain treatment in our country.

It's with some disappointment (but also optimism, because books like this continue to be published—and hopefully widely read) that I add, with minimal changes, this paragraph I wrote in a foreword for a book published over a decade ago, in 1996: "It is my hope that as you read this text, you will consider your musculoskeletal pains, and that this will encourage you to further educate yourself, as well as investigate prevention and conservative treatments, rather than rushing to take medication or subject yourself to surgery. In addition, you, the consumer of medical care, can have a positive influence on the greater medical community, helping it look more toward this type of preventive, conservative therapy to resolve one of the greatest banes of our existence—chronic pain."

—Dr. Bernard Filner, MD
   Rockville, Maryland

Preface

Every week we meet at least one new patient who has tried everything and still lives with pain that started years before. Such patients have often begun to accept a life of pain without much hope of recovery. But, in most cases, we've been able to help them substantially reduce or eliminate the pain so they can resume a normal life. It's tremendously gratifying to be able to perform this service, yet it's a continuing mystery to us that so many patients and their physicians are unaware that myofascial trigger points exist. Such patients have typically pursued other approaches to pain relief, including drugs or even surgery, without success. When they come to us, we teach them about myofascial trigger point therapy and self-care, something they have never considered.

Late in her life, Dr. Janet Travell, the pioneer of myofascial trigger point therapy, encouraged Sharon to write a book for both the general public and hands-on therapists to help them learn more about trigger points and referred pain patterns. After working together for more than ten years, we (Sharon and Mary) now feel ready to take on that task. Working together, we've been able to teach thousands of people how to lead pain-free lives. We know this book will enable us to reach out and help many we cannot treat with our own hands.

Acknowledgments

We deeply appreciate the consent of Dr. David Simons and his publisher, Wolters Kluwer Health/Lippincott Williams and Wilkins for the use of muscle and pain pattern illustrations from *Myofascial Pain and Dysfunction: The Trigger Point Manual*, volumes 1 and 2. Illustrations by Barbara D. Cummings.

We acknowledge the physicians, practitioners, and researchers who, as members of the International Myopain Society and the American Academy of Pain Management, continue to conduct important research in the field of myofascial pain and dysfunction.

We greatly appreciate our fellow myofascial trigger point therapists and others who use these techniques to relieve pain daily. And to those practitioners we have had the privilege to work with over the years, we also appreciate learning and sharing this work with you.

We are grateful to past and present students of our Myo Seminar Series. We appreciate their dedication and interest in myofascial trigger point therapy, and we've enjoyed sharing our knowledge with you. Get on out there and change the world of pain—don't manage it, get rid of it!

We also appreciate the opportunity to serve our patients. We enjoy this work. One of the great satisfactions you can have is to be able to help another person resume a normal life without pain. The basic point of this book is to show that you, the person experiencing pain, can be in charge of your own recovery, as so often happens in our clinical experience.

Thanks to Toby Lindo for his undying support during the writing of this book. Thanks also to our superb illustrator, Amanda Rose. Your organization, good spirits, and sheer talent helped us convey all we wanted to say through illustrations.

Mary: Thanks to my husband of twenty years, Mike; my daughters, Gina and Ann Marie; my siblings; and my dad. Your help and support allowed me to see this great project to completion. Lastly, to my mom. You inspired and encouraged me to follow my heart. I know you are watching over me.

Sharon: I'm happy to have been part of the Bonnie Prudden School from 1982 through 1984. When I graduated and moved to Chicago, I felt prepared to take on the world. Thanks also to my husband, Toby; my daughter, Mareva; my son, Mark; my grandchildren; and my wonder dog, Benji, who gave both Mary and me equal time during the writing of this book. And every so often, he would remind us how important it is to stop and stretch the muscles!

Introduction

When you say, "My back went out," everything in your life is put on hold. Lots of emotions flood in: disappointment, fear, anger that it happened at all or happened again, stress over loss of work and income, and more. Many questions come up: What did I do to make this happen? Why me? Why now?

As certified myofascial trigger point therapists, we call this kind of pain an *acute muscular activation*. Actually, the episode was not entirely caused by you bending, twisting, and reaching to pick up a piece of paper on the floor (or whatever innocuous event preceded the episode). In all probability, it was the accumulation of many factors. Often it's due to a lack of muscular flexibility caused by an old injury or lack of movement through the full range of motion. In addition, too much sitting can cause some muscles to overlengthen and others to shorten. Poor nutrition, poor hydration, mental or physical stress, or unaccustomed muscle use can all cause trigger point activation as well, leading to sudden, excruciating back pain

In fact, most of us harbor latent trigger points that are ready to play their part in back pain. Back pain episodes can be chronic or acute, but what they all have in common is problematic muscles—muscles designed to be used, stretched, strengthened, and lengthened. Often we ignore everyday small aches and pains and slight losses of muscular function. If left untreated, the trigger points sending these signals can cause full-blown episodes of muscle pain. Dysfunctional muscles are most often the primary cause of pain in the low back and buttocks.

Each pain problem can usually be traced to just a few muscles. If we listen to the complaint, observe and test the restrictions, and compare these findings to the information provided by Drs. Travell and Simons, the source muscles are easy to locate. Here are a few examples.

A woman sits all day at work and has a two-hour commute. One day she realizes she has pain running up and down her spine and she can't stand up straight. The problem is a chronically shortened iliopsoas muscle.

A man has difficulty bending forward and bringing his foot up and over the opposite knee to put on his socks and shoes. In this case, the problem is the gluteal (buttocks) muscles. Trigger points in these muscles can restrict forward bending while seated, and the ability to cross the legs.

A man has difficulty and pain bending down to pet his dog. In this case, the problems include trigger points and tightness in the calf muscles (soleus), the backs of the thighs (hamstrings), the buttocks (gluteal muscles), and the muscles in his back (paraspinals).

A woman has difficulty getting up from a low couch. She sits all day at work and sits again to watch TV at night. She has pain in her buttocks and around her waist. She drinks six cups of coffee a day, eats only one meal, and drinks perhaps half a glass of water each day. She tires easily and her legs feel weak. Her poor diet and sedentary lifestyle have paved the way for trigger points in her iliopsoas, gluteal muscles, and hamstrings, which also cause her feeling of general weakness.

A woman sits all day at work but can never get comfortable. She always feels she's leaning to one side and often sits on one foot until it falls asleep. She has a constant burning pain in her low back and upper buttocks and has episodes two to three times per year when her pain is so severe that she can't stand up and has to crawl to the bathroom. In this case, the problem stems from trigger points in the quadratus lumborum, a muscle in the lower back and waist, probably due to a pelvis that is smaller on one side than the other, a structural imbalance that affects her seated posture. This condition has gone undiscovered all her life. A simple change could eliminate her pain completely—if only she understood the root cause of her problem.

A man has a hard time bending down and getting into his car. He wears his belt tight around his waist and often takes long driving trips. He has pain running across his low back near his upper buttocks and can't sleep on his back anymore because of the pain. In this case, the problem is trigger points in his abdominal muscles. Yes, muscles in your abdomen can cause severe pain in the low back and upper buttocks.

When any of these muscles harbor trigger points, they can refer pain to other muscles. Those muscles in turn become activated, setting off a cascade of pain. In some instances, people end up flat on their back, unable to move, and in excruciating pain.

If any of these cases sound like your own, keep reading.

Trigger Point Therapy Can Help

According to the National Institute of Neurological Disorders and Stroke (part of the National Institutes of Health), "Americans spend over $50 billion each year on low back pain, the most common cause of job-related disability… Back pain is the second most common neurological ailment in the United States—only headache is more common" (National Institute of Neurological Disorders 2008).

Chronic low back pain (defined as lasting more than three months) can leave you tired, depressed, irritable, and hoping that somehow it will just go away. When it persists long enough, the choices sometimes seem to narrow down to either drugs or surgery. And with those choices, there are risks: drug dependency or complications due to surgery, the latter so common there's a name for it in the medical literature—*failed back surgery syndrome*, or *post-laminectomy syndrome*. If you've done your homework, you know about these conventional treatment choices and their consequences. Perhaps you've already experienced them.

While the techniques outlined in this book won't work for everyone, a majority of people who use them will experience substantial pain relief. Many of the patients we've treated successfully even had protruding or slipped disks; some had functional scoliosis or sciatic nerve pain; and some were scheduled for surgery. For these patients, locating and treating chronically contracted muscles containing trigger points turned out to be the answer.

Our patients are able to play an important part in their own recovery because we teach them self-care treatment and movement protocols. This book is intended to extend this knowledge beyond our clinic to people we cannot otherwise reach.

This book can help you become pain free and fully functional again. The most important factor will be *your* persistence and hard work. You'll also need to build a kit of inexpensive self-care tools you'll learn about in chapter 3. A combination of the right tools, a better understanding of muscular pain, and diligence in performing self-care can help you eliminate your pain and prevent episodes of back pain from recurring.

The Origins of Myofascial Trigger Point Therapy

The seminal works in the field of myofascial trigger point therapy are two big books entitled *Myofascial Pain and Dysfunction: The Trigger Point Manual* (volumes 1 and 2). First published in 1983 and 1992, these books are still the best technical resources in the field. They were coauthored by Janet Travell, MD, the first female personal physician to the president (John Kennedy), and David Simons, MD. They wrote about the basic causes of chronic myofascial pain (soft tissue pain), the reason for one-third of all doctor visits in the United States, something costing untold billions of dollars every year for testing, drugs, surgery, psychotherapy, and countless protocols for dealing with pain that run the gamut from exotic to mundane. Based on our combined thirty-five years of clinical experience using the techniques described in these books, we believe Travell and Simons came close to finding the gold standard for treating myofascial pain, including low back pain.

Unfortunately, their work has had little impact on the way pain is treated today. Their methods have received little attention in medical schools, and their work is rarely cited in mainstream medical literature. Of 3,600 citations on low back pain between 1996 and 2002, only 0.5 percent were also indexed under myofascial trigger points or just trigger points. The percentage never reached 1 percent in any single year. However, the majority of cases of low back pain are caused by myofascial trigger points (Simons 2004).

Most physicians are unfamiliar with muscular referred pain patterns or methods used to eliminate them, such as trigger point pressure release. Few physicians are sufficiently informed about them to offer or prescribe treatment or give a referral to a practitioner qualified to perform it. In addition, there aren't that many trained myofascial trigger point therapists or ancillary health care providers adequately trained in this work. We are working to remedy this situation by conducting our ongoing Myo Seminar Series, one of the few trigger point therapy training programs in the world based on Travell and Simons's work (see www.myopain.com).

It's stunning to contrast our daily experience of treating and relieving pain for people who have suffered severe, long-lasting pain problems with the reality that the medical profession is largely unaware of the whole phenomenon and often leads people to believe they have to live with their pain for the rest of their lives. In sum, Travell and Simons described methods that work, and often work spectacularly, but are all too rarely used.

Dr. Travell wrote her first paper on trigger points in 1942. She continued to work to the end of her life, in 1997, at the age of ninety-six. I (Sharon) first met her in 1986 and assisted her at a number of workshops in the late 1980s and early 1990s. We spoke often about her work, and once I got up the nerve to ask her why she didn't include more information about hands-on treatment in her books. She said,

"Doctors are trained to use needles. A hands-on myofascial trigger point therapy book—that's for you to write." That was the genesis for this book.

Why Isn't Trigger Point Therapy Better Known?

We've often tried to account for the almost total lack of attention myofascial trigger points receive in the medical field—despite the fact that every day we perform therapy that relieves chronic pain in the great majority of people coming to us.

We've had many patients who were scheduled for surgery but after being treated with trigger point elimination techniques, chose not to go through with surgery because their pain was gone. We've also treated people who had already undergone surgery. Some of them qualified for the diagnosis of failed back surgery syndrome. Although pain relief is more difficult in such cases, we are usually able to help. Additionally, general anesthetic and surgical procedures sometimes activate latent trigger points, so we often treat painful conditions caused or exacerbated by surgery.

Myofascial trigger point therapy doesn't require complex or expensive equipment. In fact, trigger point therapy is pretty low-tech. And although an X-ray or MRI won't confirm the presence of chronic myofascial pain, hundreds of thousands of them are done every year just to conclude that "there's nothing wrong with you." In short, drug companies and purveyors of high-tech medical equipment have little incentive to invest in research confirming the efficacy of myofascial trigger point therapy. Of course, without such research, many physicians are understandably reluctant to recommend it.

And it's hard for doctors who've already given seven years or more to the study of medicine to devote more time to a new, somewhat complex field. Plus, the economics of the medical profession, with enormous overhead and insurance burdens, pretty much rules out an approach to pain treatment that can take an hour or more to perform.

Given these considerations, it's often easier to prescribe drugs or even surgery for serious pain problems. Even though there's limited research to back up the efficacy of surgery for chronic back pain, drugs and surgery are usually deemed "reasonable and customary," the magic words that guarantee bills sent to your insurance company get paid.

Since the early 1950s, U.S. medical costs have gone from 4 percent to over 15 percent of our gross domestic product, and the percentage is projected to climb higher as the population continues to age (California HealthCare Foundation 2008). Since back pain is the second most common affliction prompting visits to physicians, it accounts for a substantial share of this vast financial drain.

At times it seems a daunting task for us to bring myofascial trigger point therapy into the mainstream of pain treatment. Too many things seem stacked against it. But a look at the history of medicine in the United States gives grounds for hope. Only sixty years ago, physicians were still doing lobotomies. Today, quite a few physicians recognize the dangers of surgery and drug dependency and the possibly damaging side effects of drugs, and they are more cautious in recommending surgery or prescribing medications. Perhaps some in mainstream medicine will embrace myofascial trigger point therapy as a low-tech approach to preventing and treating chronic low back pain and many other pain conditions all over the body. In the meantime, you can learn how to do it yourself using this book.

Trigger Point Therapy—Safe and Effective Relief

Among the millions suffering from low back pain, many are willing to take a hand in their own recovery. And thousands of gifted health care practitioners have a good working knowledge of muscular anatomy, making them an ideal fit to use trigger point techniques in their work. This book is intended as a resource for both the general public and practitioners who treat muscular pain in the low back and buttocks.

Myofascial trigger point therapy is a prudent option because it's a conservative form of treatment. Once your doctor has ruled out cancer or other life-threatening causes of pain, there's little risk or downside to trying myofascial trigger point therapy. Unlike surgery or drugs, there are no lasting side effects. If it doesn't work you can try another method. And if it does work, you've got your life back! For this reason alone, myofascial trigger point therapy should be an early option, not a last resort.

Who We Are, and Why We Wrote This Book

Sharon's Story

I learned about trigger point therapy back in 1982 when I had migraine headaches I couldn't shake. I found a myotherapist (what we now call a myofascial trigger point therapist) in Amherst, Massachusetts. After one treatment, I was so impressed I visited the school she had attended, founded by Bonnie Prudden in nearby Lenox, Massachusetts. During that visit I signed up for two years of training, even though the fall term had already started! When I began my training, I knew nothing about physical fitness, exercise, trigger points, or hands-on treatment.

Bonnie Prudden is a great teacher who developed the field of hands-on myotherapy based on research done by Drs. Travell and Simons. A renowned fitness instructor, she was also one of the founders of the President's Council on Physical Fitness in the 1950s. She helped raise awareness of poor fitness levels in the United States and has written over thirty books on physical fitness and myofascial pain treatment.

Before finding myofascial trigger point therapy, I was an artist and musician. Since learning myofascial trigger point therapy, I've devoted my life to pain relief. Although I spent most of the 1970s and early 1980s in other parts of the country, after learning myofascial trigger point therapy I returned to my hometown of Chicago in 1986. I've had a full-time clinical practice in Chicago ever since. Over the past twenty-two years I've treated thousands of people from almost every state and several foreign countries. I've also served as director of treatment and training for five pain clinics in greater Chicago.

In my training programs on myofascial trigger point therapy, I've taught hundreds of others these pain relief techniques. I first met one of those trainees as a patient in 1998. Her name was Mary Biancalana.

Mary's Story

I've enjoyed working for twenty-four years in fitness and health education. My fascination with muscles, their function, their problems, their influence on posture, and how to help athletes remain pain free and in top form led me to study and coach people in all types of activities. My bachelor's degree in physical education and masters in education have supported my work in teaching others fitness concepts as well as trigger point therapy in our MYO Seminar Series. As a myofascial trigger point therapist and certified personal trainer, I've served as director of therapy and director of self-care training for two pain clinics in greater Chicago.

I first learned about myofascial trigger point therapy because of a car accident that left me with pain in my neck and upper back. A friend referred me to Sharon Sauer. From my first treatment in 1998, I knew trigger point therapy would change my life, and I soon began to study and practice in this field. And because of my background as a personal trainer, I've been able to help develop and expand the self-care training protocols used to support our clinical treatment and our training seminars.

I'm particularly interested in how structural problems contribute to chronic pain, including low back pain. Many of our patients have suffered for a long time with undiagnosed structural problems such as Morton's foot syndrome, hyperpronation, a small *hemipelvis* (one sit bone smaller than the other), or uneven leg length. These problems often turn out to be the principal perpetuating factors in their pain, and correcting them can profoundly change people's lives. In chapter 17, we'll show you how to test for and correct such conditions.

Working Together

Since we have each been affected, both personally and professionally, by trigger point therapy, we've strived to train as many practitioners as possible. There's plenty of pain to go around. Sharon has been teaching these techniques since 1989, and since 2000, we've worked together to train doctors, dentists, chiropractors, physical therapists, massage therapists, nurses, acupuncturists, other health care professionals, and personal trainers through our Myo Seminar Series. Together, we have been featured speakers at many conferences and symposiums, not only for medical practitioners interested in trigger point therapy, but also for the general public.

Both health care practitioners and the general population are becoming more aware of trigger points and referred pain, and how to treat them. The most distinctive feature of our practice is how we empower our patients with education in self-care treatment. We give all of them self-care protocol sheets outlining the muscles most likely to be causing their pain, and we teach them how to perform self-care for those areas.

Because of the nature of their work, many health care professionals are prone to chronic low back pain. That's why self-care is essential for practitioners as well as the general public. And that's another reason we've written this book for both.

How to Use This Book

This book is focused on the myofascial component of pain in the low back and buttocks and the symptoms and referred pain patterns associated with trigger points responsible for that pain. You'll learn how to alleviate your own low back pain through self-evaluation and a self-care treatment protocol combining warm-up, compression, stretching (in combination with contracting and relaxing), and movement. And learning how to treat your own trigger points can be fun, empowering, and vastly rewarding.

Learning the Basics

The first three chapters give you an overview of trigger points and treatment techniques. In chapter 1, you'll learn what trigger points are, how to find them, and what causes them. You'll also learn about the phenomenon of referred pain and why you must look for the cause of your pain in places other than where you feel the pain.

In chapter 2, you'll learn how to apply compression, how hard to apply it, how often, in what position, and so on. We'll discuss how and when to use heat and cold as part of treatment. You'll learn why movement and stretching are essential to effective therapy. You'll also gain an understanding of the feedback loops involved in muscular pain. This will allow you to read the signals your body is sending you so you'll know when you're on the right track with the self-care techniques you're using.

In chapter 3, we'll discuss the various self-care tools you'll need to accomplish your goals. If you're determined to relieve your pain, it makes sense to acquire a modest kit of self-care tools that will vastly improve your results. You'll learn about compression therapy balls, the Backnobber, the Jacknobber, Fomentek bags, Mother Earth Pillows, stretching straps, foam rollers, and more. You'll learn how to use each tool and how these tools can make self-treatment something you look forward to.

The Muscle Chapters: A Road Map to Pain Relief

Chapter 4 provides a comprehensive index of symptoms associated with low back and buttocks pain. Each symptom is a clue to the most likely muscle (or muscles) causing your pain. As you look through the index, check off the symptoms that best describe the specific pain or dysfunction you're experiencing. After each symptom, you'll see a reference to the specific muscle or muscles associated with that symptom. You can use chapter 4 as a road map to the muscle chapters you'll need to study in depth.

Chapters 5 through 15 address each of the muscles that can either cause or refer pain to the low back and buttocks. (Some chapters include more than one muscle.) We've arranged the muscle chapters by how frequently they cause low back pain: iliopsoas, paraspinals, rectus abdominis, quadratus lumborum, the gluteal muscles (including the gluteus maximus, medius, and minimus and the piriformis), hamstrings, soleus, and the pelvic floor muscles.

In each of the muscle chapters, you'll learn where the muscle is, what it does, where to look for trigger points, and the referred pain patterns associated with trigger points in that muscle. You'll also learn specific compression techniques, stretches, and contractions to help relieve your pain and restore the muscles to full function. Self-care for all the buttock muscles—the gluteus maximus, gluteus medius, gluteus minimus, and piriformis—involves very similar techniques, so we've chosen to cover all aspects of buttocks treatment in chapter 12. The muscle chapters are well illustrated so you can see all aspects of self-care. You may need to practice the positions shown in these illustrations to fully understand the techniques.

Based on the sections of the muscle chapters titled "Do I Have Trigger Points in My…" and the simple range of motion tests these sections include, you can determine which muscles have trigger points and dysfunction. You may find you only need to carefully study three or four muscle chapters to address the specific problems causing your back pain. But there's no harm in reading every chapter. And if you're a health care practitioner, careful study of every muscle chapter is essential.

Each muscle chapter also contains more detailed information for health care practitioners at the end, under "For Practitioners." These sections describe how to use this book in clinical practice, including how to more thoroughly evaluate and treat myofascial pain, and things to avoid in dealing with it. They also cover more complex range of motion testing and how to deal with severe pain problems. We encourage practitioners to use this book as a resource to teach patients how to take an active role in their own recovery. Professional guidance can make all the difference in helping people overcome years of chronic pain and dysfunction. This book offers an effective alternative to the standard treatments for back pain: proven self-care methods that work better than painkillers or surgery in many cases.

Other Aspects of Trigger Point Therapy

In the last two chapters of the book, we address more general but critically important aspects of myofascial trigger point therapy. In chapter 16, Range of Motion Exercises, we describe and illustrate movement exercises for all the muscles that refer pain to the low back. These movement exercises are essential to full recovery and maintaining a pain-free life.

In chapter 17, General Perpetuating Factors, we address important structural and systemic problems that can play a critical part in low back pain but often go undetected. We teach you how to perform simple screenings for such perpetuating factors as structural problems of the feet, legs, or pelvis and poor posture when sitting, sleeping, or standing. We also touch on other conditions that can cause, magnify, or perpetuate pain.

Contraindications for Myofascial Trigger Point Treatment

The recommendations in this book are based on the assumption that you've consulted your primary care physician about your low back pain, and possibly specialists, as well. If you haven't done so, we urge you to take that step first, as there are many possible causes of persistent back pain that are nonmyofascial in origin. For example, one cause of chronic low back pain could be kidney stones or blockages.

The responsibility properly rests with your doctor to determine whether your pain has a possibly serious nonmyofascial cause. Assuming your physician has ruled out all such causes, certain medical conditions make it inadvisable to undergo myofascial trigger point treatment. Among those for whom such treatment may not be recommended are people with malignant tumors, those taking blood thinners such as warfarin (Coumadin), and those with severe osteoporosis or arteriosclerosis.

Also, special care should be exercised in the treatment of people who have had hip replacement, spinal fusion, spinal decompression, or a diskectomy. People who have had any of these operations should follow the recommendations in this book *only with the approval of their personal physician*, and should carefully respect any limitations their physician may prescribe.

Getting Started

So you're ready to dig in, right? There's just one more subject we'd like to introduce to you: Let's talk about who you are, what your starting point is, what your goal is, and how much effort you're willing to devote. After all, we're not offering a quick fix, but rather an ongoing approach to keeping your muscles healthy.

Who Are You and What Is Your Starting Point?

The recommendations in this book need to be adjusted based on your age, fitness level, general health, flexibility, severity of pain, and so on. Please begin by making an honest survey of your starting point, and then think about how to adjust our self-care protocols to respect it. For example, if you're in nearly unbearable pain, you'll need more gentle, more frequent, and probably more prolonged treatment than if your pain is intermittent and mild. Your age can also affect the time it takes to heal. In general, the older you are and the longer you've been living with pain, the longer it will take to reach a pain-free state and full function. If you're in excellent health, you'll need less time to normalize your muscles and become pain free. If you're overweight, sedentary, drink too much alcohol, have irregular sleeping habits, smoke, or have limited range of motion in much of your body, recovery will take longer and you'll need to make significant adjustments to your lifestyle in order to reduce your pain and restore full function.

If your pain is myofascial in origin, as it is with most cases of acute or chronic low back and buttocks pain, maybe only two or three muscles contain active trigger points and are severely dysfunctional. However, it would be unusual to find the rest of your muscles in tip-top condition. The reality is that even if most of your muscles work acceptably, many will contain at least latent trigger points and have some limitation of range of motion. You probably aren't aware of these potential problems because they don't significantly affect your day-to-day activities and you've become adapted to the limitations they impose. Those limitations come about gradually, and are easily misinterpreted as just one more sign that you're getting older.

So you can limit your use of this book to locating and treating those (relatively few) muscles containing active trigger points, that is, those primarily responsible for your referred pain. Or you can take time to read the whole book and get to know a great deal about the anatomy and potential perpetuating factors affecting the low back. That way you'll have the knowledge you need for a more comprehensive program of self-care to help you stay pain free in the long run.

What's Your Goal?

Do you want to just get rid of the pain you're feeling right now? Or do you want to get rid of that pain, correct underlying perpetuating factors, *and* prevent a recurrence of pain for the foreseeable future? There's a difference between these goals. The first can usually be achieved within a few weeks if you're persistent and dedicated. The second may take a little time every day for the rest of your life. In this, as in most other aspects of life, you get what you pay for—or what you put into it.

We don't want to bully you into a particular goal. Our purpose is to help you reach your goal, whatever it is. But we can offer you a more complete guide to life without low back pain if you're willing to make self-care a part of your life on an ongoing basis.

Keep Working on It

At this point, you may view this book with some skepticism, especially if you've tried all manner of tests and treatments in a fruitless search for some relief. But please keep an open mind and a willing heart as you study the information we offer. And look for the small changes you'll soon feel, in pain, function, or range of motion, that tell you something is happening to your body. Although these improvements are sometimes small at the outset, this is how your recovery will start!

It's strange that the majority of low back pain is caused by myofascial trigger points (Simons 2004), and yet modern medicine treats the subject of trigger points mostly with silence. How could the answer be so simple, and so completely overlooked? Could the answer to your pain be in your hands now? Could it be as simple as locating and treating active trigger points yourself?

Yes, it could. The path usually isn't a straight line from beginning to the pain-free end. But remember, this isn't another way to mask the pain, as with drugs. This is a way to find the root cause of the pain and eliminate it.

When you've made it through to the end and achieved your goal, we hope to hear from you. We'll be happy for your success, but not surprised. We only ask that you share the story of your success with others who might benefit from this approach. Tell them about this book. We hope it will help them as much as it helped you.

Chapter 1

Trigger Points and Referred Pain Patterns

Throughout this book we use the term *myofascial*, so let's start with the definition of that term. *Myo* is Greek for "muscle," and *fascia*, as defined by the 2007 Fascia Research Congress, is "the soft tissue… [that] interpenetrates and surrounds muscles, bones, organs, nerves, blood vessels, and other structures. Fascia is an uninterrupted, three-dimensional web of tissue that extends from head to toe, from front to back, from interior to exterior. [It] provides the matrix that allows for intercellular communication" (Fascia Research Congress 2007). So in a broader sense, "myofascial" applies to all soft tissue, including the muscles, tendons, ligaments, and even the skin. Although we discuss myofascial pain throughout this book largely in terms of dysfunctional muscles, it may help you to know that it's also possible to treat and eliminate trigger points in tendons and ligaments.

Some Basic Anatomy

Before discussing trigger points and referred pain patterns, let's begin with some basic anatomy so that you'll be familiar with the muscles and bones we discuss in this book.

Muscles

In this book, we cover ten muscles or muscle groups that can cause low back or buttock pain when they contain active trigger points.

Iliopsoas. This muscle is located deep within the abdomen and hip. It connects the lumbar vertebrae and the iliac crest to the top of the femur (thigh bone). It helps raise the thigh (hip flexion) or brings the chest to the thigh. If you sit most of the time, this keeps the muscle shortened. It may be the single most overlooked muscle in the body in terms of probable cause for low back pain.

Paraspinals. This muscle group consists of both superficial muscles (the erector spinae) and deeper muscles (multifidi and rotatores) that control rotational and bending movements of the torso. The long superficial muscles run up and down parallel to the spine; the deeper muscles are much shorter and run diagonally between the vertebrae. The superficial group stabilizes the torso and helps with bending forward and backward and coming back to a neutral posture. The deeper group rotates the spine and, when dysfunctional, can contribute to such phenomena as bulging or compressed disks and nerve compression along the spine.

Rectus abdominis. This muscle is the focus in the search for "six-pack" abs. It runs up and down over the abdomen, between the lowest ribs and the top of the pubic bone. It helps stabilize the torso.

Gluteus maximus. This is the most superficial and by far the largest of the gluteal muscles. It forms the largest part of the buttocks and works to bring the thigh back (hip extension), so it has a function opposite that of the iliopsoas muscle.

Gluteus medius and minimus. These muscles lie beneath the gluteus maximus in layers, the medius being more superficial and the minimus being deeper. They act to rotate the thigh and swing the leg out to the side. It's best to treat them together, as they are so close it can be difficult to distinguish one from the other.

Piriformis. This cigar-shaped muscle lies deep within the buttocks and connects the thigh bone to the pelvis near the sacrum. It's primarily responsible for rotating the thigh outward and for swinging the leg out to the side when the hip is flexed. Trigger points in this muscle can entrap the sciatic nerve.

Quadratus lumborum. Deeper within the sides of the torso, roughly covering the area of the kidneys, this muscle can act alone to bend the torso to the side or rotate it. Acting together with the superficial paraspinals, it helps with straightening the torso up after bending forward. Like the iliopsoas, it's one of the most commonly overlooked sources of low back pain, and when dysfunctional it can cause some of the most excruciating pain a person can experience.

Hamstrings. Most people have had a hamstring "pull" at some time. This isn't actually a snapped or pulled muscle, but a cramping or contraction of the muscle caused by activation of trigger points, usually due to putting the muscle in shortened position, such as while sitting, and trying to run while it's still shortened. These long muscles run along the back of the thigh from the sit bones in the buttocks down to the top of the tibia, one of the bones in the lower leg. The hamstrings help bend the knee and stabilize the thigh at the knee.

Soleus. Of all muscles covered in this book, the soleus, located deep in the calf, is the farthest from the low back. This muscle is a strong plantar flexor (helps us go up on our "tiptoes") and contributes to knee and ankle stability. When dysfunctional, it is a primary cause of heel pain. When trigger points in the lower outside region of this muscle become activated, it refers pain all the way to the area around the sacrum at the base of the spine.

Pelvic floor muscles. These muscles form the bottom of the abdomen and create a sling that holds the abdominal organs in place at the base of the pelvis. Because of their location, they can be difficult to treat and are often overlooked as a possible cause of low back pain.

Bones

Keep in mind that bones don't move themselves; muscles move bones and nerves move muscles. When muscles are dysfunctional, they can contribute to misalignment (as in functional scoliosis, which is often caused by chronic shortening of the muscles in the torso), bulging or protruding disks, and even bone spurs. Believe it or not, over time when muscular dysfunction is corrected, X-rays and MRIs often confirm that misalignment has been lessened or eliminated, bulging disks decompress, and bone spurs reabsorb. It is for these reasons that we urge you to consider a muscular origin or solution to your pain. Let's take a look at the more important bone structures involved in low back pain.

Vertebrae. These bones, which make up the spinal column, are divided into four sections named for their location along the spine. There are seven *cervical* vertebrae, located at the very top of the spine, in the neck and base of the skull; twelve *thoracic* vertebrae, in the area of the chest; five *lumbar* vertebrae, running behind the abdomen; and the *sacrum*, at the base of the spine, which consists of five vertebrae that are fused together (four in the *coccyx*, or tailbone, and a final segment at the very bottom of the spine). Each vertebra is an incredibly complex and delicate structure that provides for various muscle attachments, the passage of the spinal cord, and openings for nerves to enter and exit (the *foramen*). The vertebrae are sturdy and strong; however, they are the most at risk of developing osteoporosis and compression fractures as we get older. Good nutrition and exercise go hand in hand with protecting our spines. The *spinous process* is the part of the spine you can feel if you bend over at the waist and run your hand over your spine. The *transverse processes* are the "wings" that extend to either side of the vertebrae. Trigger points in the muscles that attach to the vertebrae at any point along the spine can cause severe pain and dysfunction. When dysfunctional muscles pull the vertebrae closer together, they can cause true nerve root compression; however, proper treatment can release the trigger points and relieve the nerve root compression.

Pelvis. The pelvic structure consists of three basic elements: the *pubic symphysis* (the bony mass at the bottom of the abdomen, the *iliac crest* (the large fan-shaped bones that form the structure of the buttocks); and the *ischial tuberosities* (often called the *sit bones*, as these are the bones we sit on). The gluteal muscles, quadratus lumborum, paraspinals, piriformis, pelvic floor muscles, and hamstrings all attach to some part of the pelvic structure.

Femur. This is the large thigh bone, the head of which fits into the acetabulum, or socket of the pelvis. It has many bumps or protuberances. Two of these protuberances are important for us to consider: the lesser trochanter is a small protuberance on the inner surface of the femur, to which the iliopsoas attaches, and the greater trochanter, a large protuberance, is where several important muscles such as gluteus medius, gluteus minimus, and the piriformis attach.

Causes of Low Back Pain

With low back pain, the first thing to do is see your doctor. Due to the proximity of the abdominal organs, low back pain can originate in the internal organs themselves. In fact, there can be a reciprocal influence between the internal organs and the muscles. Problems with the organs can activate trigger points in the muscles, resulting in pain and muscle dysfunction. Conversely, muscular trigger points can cause the organs to have numerous problems (Simons, Travell, and Simons 1999, p. 959).

An example of low back pain originating in the organs is when the renal system (the kidneys and renal tubes) becomes inflamed or distended. In this condition, the affected kidney can refer pain to the same side of the low back. Gallstones can also cause severe low back pain, and contraction of the uterus during menstruation or childbirth can cause strong pain in the abdomen and low back. If your doctor has ruled out organ problems as the source of your pain but you don't achieve any significant improvement in your pain levels using the self-care treatments described in this book (including addressing any perpetuating factors noted in chapter 17), we recommend you visit your doctor again and request more extensive testing.

Interestingly, in many cases muscular dysfunction can cause or exacerbate other conditions thought to originate in the internal organs, including severe menstrual cramps, colic in babies, anorexia, nausea, diarrhea, bladder dysfunction, heartburn, indigestion, vomiting, and irritable bowel syndrome (Simons, Travell, and Simons 1999, pp. 943, 958). There are also several joints in and around the area of the low back and buttocks that could be contributing to your pain. Travell and Simons point out that most general practitioners lack adequate training and skills to determine whether joint dysfunction is a possible cause of pain. You may need to consult an MD specializing in physiatry, orthopedics, radiology, or neurology, or an osteopath, physical therapist, or chiropractor to determine whether joint problems are the root cause of your pain.

Clearly, persistent pain can be a sign of many different medical conditions, some of them quite serious. But if you've already checked out those possibilities and they've been ruled out, yet your pain persists, then what?

Two very common recommendations given by many health care providers are rest and a mild pain reliever, and then stronger pain medications if the first one doesn't help. If you have a chronic pain condition (for our purposes meaning lasting more than three months), you've probably tried those approaches already. If that had worked, you wouldn't be reading this book. If myofascial trigger points are causing your pain, be aware that they don't go away on their own, and they certainly don't yield to pain relievers and bed rest. In fact, masking the pain with medication can often make the underlying condition worse. And because movement is essential for releasing trigger points, bed rest can actually be counterproductive, as well.

The Problem with Standard Treatment Approaches

To us, it seems simple: If there are trigger points in the muscle tissue and you're experiencing pain and other problems as a result, don't mask the problems, and don't stop using the muscles because you have pain—fix them! Unfortunately, the pain clinic approach often seems to consist of medicating the pain without ever getting to the source of the problem: the muscles themselves and the posture or habits of the person whose body they reside in. If the problem is dysfunctional muscular tissues, it doesn't make sense to mask the pain with drugs, talk to a counselor about it, remove various body parts or tissues

Latent Trigger Points

As you might imagine, *latent trigger points* are those that aren't currently active. For example, you might have sustained a childhood injury many years ago that left you with trigger points that haven't caused pain for years. Most of us probably have quite a few latent trigger points scattered around our muscles. You won't be aware of them, because latent trigger points don't make much of a fuss at all unless you press on them or challenge the muscles that contain them.

However, they are sites for potential problems down the road. Various factors, including nutritional deficiencies, postural imbalances, breathing problems, and physical stress, can cause those latent trigger points to activate, causing a real pain problem—perhaps like the one you're living with right now. Once you've deactivated the trigger points that are causing the referred pain you feel, you may believe you've solved the problem and can go back to business as usual. However, some ongoing self-care will be helpful in preventing latent trigger points from becoming active and bringing you to your knees once again.

Other Kinds of Trigger Points

Central trigger points are either active or latent. They occur where the motor nerves innervate the muscle. These motor nerves provide the communication that tells the muscle to contract. Central trigger points and the taut bands of tissue containing them must be released to eliminate attachment trigger points.

Attachment trigger points occur at the attachment of the muscle tendon to the bone, and also where the muscle merges into the tendon. Attachment trigger points can cause pain and swelling at the attachment to the bone, which is usually called tendinitis. To get rid of "tendinitis," you need to eliminate the central trigger point and the taut band, as this is the cause of tension at the tendon/bone attachment.

A *key trigger point* can activate trigger points in other muscles within the area of its referral pattern; these are known as *satellite trigger points*. Deactivation of key trigger points can stop satellite trigger points from reactivating; however, satellite trigger points may still require direct treatment.

A Holistic View

Dysfunctional muscle tissue feels different than healthy tissue. When palpating such tissue, you notice a definite hardness or tension in the tissue that isn't present in healthy muscles. The area of palpable dysfunction can vary in size depending on the muscle and the severity of the problem. You often notice that the tissue isn't supple. And in areas where circulation is severely compromised, the tissue tends to remain slightly depressed after being compressed. We call this *myofascial pitting* and consider it to be a definite indicator that the area needs treatment.

Normal muscle tissue is constantly being nourished through blood circulation. Movement fosters this process of replenishment, so when normal movement takes place daily, the muscles can maintain healthy tone and local circulation. But when movement is limited, as it almost always is with pain or a sedentary lifestyle, the muscles weaken, tighten, and develop trigger points and other problems. Eventually, this can cause the muscle to shut down, in a sense, resulting in a downward spiral where immobility produces more weakness and pain, and the weakness and pain cause you to move even less. And when trigger points refer pain to other areas, this cascade widens to include other muscles and other parts of the body—clearly a highly undesirable situation.

Our experience as therapists has taught us to concern ourselves with the whole muscle, not just the most contracted segments. It's better to think of trigger points as a characteristic of dysfunctional muscle tissue, rather than the entirety of the problem. If we had to choose a single all-encompassing phrase to describe the nature of trigger points, we'd say "taut bands of muscle tissue containing intensely painful areas." However, even though this is a more accurate way to describe the condition we're looking for, it's also pretty cumbersome. So throughout this book, we'll use the phrase "trigger points" to mean those taut bands of muscle tissue containing intensely painful areas.

Referred Pain Patterns

Referred pain is really the core of this book. Our goal is to help you identify which muscles are dysfunctional and then fix them so the referral of pain to your lower back and buttocks will stop. Most of the muscles we discuss are located in the back, the buttocks, the abdomen, or the thighs. But one of them, the soleus, is in the calf. How can that be? How can a muscle in the lower leg somehow transmit or refer pain to the lower back? Let's take a look at the process.

The process of pain referral from myofascial trigger points is a neurological phenomenon. The nervous system transmits a signal from the area of dysfunctional muscle tissue containing the trigger point complex back to the central nervous system. This causes pain to be felt in a pattern that is specific for that muscle. These patterns are often located somewhere in the area supplied by that muscle's nerve supply as well as other nerves located above and below that spinal segment. The signal may be felt as pain, numbness, tingling, weakness, heightened sensitivity, or loss of sensation in the referral area. Since trigger points refer pain *away* from where they are located, it is critically important that you find out what muscle harbors the primary trigger point *causing* the pain and eliminate it. It is for this reason that while many practitioners provide intervention where it hurts, the pain does not go away if it is primarily referred by myofascial trigger points located in another region of the body.

If referred pain is a big part of your lower back pain, you may wonder what you can do about it. Fortunately, there are only ten muscles or muscle groups that refer pain to the low back and buttocks. Even in the most serious cases, usually only a few of these muscles are dysfunctional. So your task isn't too difficult: Simply find and properly treat a handful of muscles that are causing the problem. The intensity and exact location of your pain will point to a few suspect muscles. The rest of this book will help you narrow your list of suspects and teach you how to do simple self-care treatment to relieve the pain those dysfunctional muscles are causing.

Strength Training and Traditional Physical Therapy

Many of our patients report that they "failed" physical therapy or that their pain and dysfunction became worse after going through a program of physical therapy. They're often angry at the doctor who referred them to physical therapy because it made them worse. Sometimes they're regarded as malingerers because they don't improve as expected. However, the approach they've been prescribed is futile for one simple reason: Their trigger points are neither identified nor treated. In such circumstances, strengthening exercises are a waste of time.

Trigger points cause muscle weakness as well as pain. If trigger points aren't deactivated, the muscle remains weak, no matter how much strengthening you do. In fact, trying to strengthen muscles with active trigger points usually intensifies both the pain and the weakness. We've encountered some weight-training enthusiasts who previously could bench press 250 pounds or more and came to us barely able to carry a grocery bag. This is what happens if you ignore pain and dysfunction and continue to try to strengthen your muscles. The first step to recovery is to deactivate trigger points and restore full range of motion. Only then should you resume strengthening. Even then, it's important to start with low weight and low reps, and to continue your self-care during training. In general, a good rule is "length equals strength." A muscle with trigger points may not fully lengthen or shorten, and for that reason it will have diminished strength and power and will fatigue more easily.

How Muscle Relaxation Relates to Muscle Health

Muscles containing trigger points can't fully relax. When muscles are chronically contracted, cellular production of energy is reduced, which perpetuates the tightness. This is where compression treatment helps. Compression, as well as stretching, contracting, and movement, tends to stimulate greater local circulation and therefore nutrient exchange, which in turn stimulates the production of energy by the cells. So compression treatment helps break the cycle of pain, tightness, and more pain so you can begin to relax your muscles.

Healthy muscles should be relaxed when they aren't in use. They should also remain relaxed when another person shortens or lengthens the muscle by putting it through its *passive range of motion*. Healthy muscles shouldn't even unconsciously "help" during a passive movement. When we assess for muscle dysfunction, we instruct the patient to remain relaxed while we move their body. If we detect this unconscious "helping," or contraction of the muscles during passive range of motion, it's a clear sign of myofascial dysfunction and underlying trigger points.

Summary

If referred pain patterns are news to you, we encourage you to think of this as good news, because it offers a way to relieve your pain you haven't yet tried. Trigger points are the source of this referred pain, and when you find them, you'll need to treat them with the techniques we describe, including compression, stretching, range of motion exercise, contracting, and relaxing. As you start self-care treatment, look for changes in your pain level and muscle flexibility. As these changes begin to occur, you'll know you're on the right track. This will help you stick with your self-care program until your pain is gone, and continue with preventive self-care to avoid a recurrence of your pain. You might want to keep a written record of changes in your pain levels, range of motion, and strength, since it can be difficult to detect changes that occur gradually.

Chapter 2

Treatment Techniques

In this chapter, we'll describe the basic elements of self-care treatment. Although compression of taut bands of muscle is at the heart of treatment, an effective self-care program also includes warming up prior to treatment; sequences of stretching, contracting, and relaxing; and gentle range of motion exercises. Like most chapters in this book, this chapter has two sections: the first for all readers, the second, located at the end, primarily for practitioners who will be applying these techniques to others.

Pain Is Information: Pay Attention to It

This book will work best if you really focus on your pain: Exactly what does it feel like? Where is it? When does it get better? When does it get worse? Is it better or worse today than yesterday? Has it moved since yesterday? Answers to these questions can help you find the muscle or muscles most likely to be causing your pain.

Subtle changes, not only from day to day, but even during your self-care treatment, can tell you whether you're on the right track. The best signal is a feeling of "hurting good." Although that expression is a bit vague and could mean different things to different people, it's a feeling we (and most patients) have when compression is applied to a spot containing trigger points. While it does involve some discomfort, it also feels good in that you're aware of a feeling of stimulation or increased sensation. You're actually sensing a subtle process of relaxation, a letting go in the tissue. This is, in fact, what actually happens as your muscle begins to regain its normal flexibility and capacity to function.

The Site of Pain vs. the Source of Pain

For trigger point compression to work, you need to press on the areas in a muscle where taut fibers and trigger points are located. If you have pain in your low back, it may seem that the low back is the area needing attention. But due to the phenomenon of referred pain, your low back pain is more likely to be caused by muscles in your abdomen, mid back, waist, or thighs, or even your lower legs. So you can treat your low back until the end of time, but if you aren't treating the *source* of the pain, it will persist. In the muscle chapters, we provide illustrations of typical referred pain patterns, lists of the most likely symptoms, and easy screening tests to help you figure out which muscles may be causing your pain. You can also narrow your search by referring to chapter 4, where we've gathered the illustrations of the referred pain patterns for the muscles covered in this book. Chapter 4 also contains a table listing many common symptoms and medical diagnoses that can be attributed to trigger points in the muscles covered in this book. Using the table in chapter 4 as a "cheat sheet," locate your symptom and use the table to determine the muscle or muscles that may be responsible for that symptom.

Keep Looking for the Source of the Pain

Sometimes it seems that when you fix one muscle, other muscles get "jealous" and send you a pain signal so they can get some of that wonderful attention. In most parts of the body there are multiple layers of muscle. When the outer layer contains trigger points and taut bands, this can mask problems in the deeper layers. And when you eliminate trigger points in the superficial layer, trigger points in the deeper muscles may become activated and require treatment as well. The point is to keep looking for painful spots and restricted range of motion, and to correct them as you detect them. This is often how the healing process unfolds. Stay with it, and recognize that any change in the nature, intensity, or location of the pain is a signal that your muscles are responding to treatment. In general, your pain will move, and over time it will get less intense and more localized before it is completely eliminated.

Why Treat an Area If It Doesn't Hurt?

Some people say, "My muscles didn't hurt until I started pressing on them—why not just leave them alone?" The answer is, you can leave them alone, but if they contain trigger points, they won't leave you alone, at least not in the long run. Muscle problems should be corrected before they turn into debilitating pain or even greater dysfunction. Perhaps you've experienced just a little weakness, a twinge of pain, or a small limitation in range of motion and have written it off as due to aging, tendonitis, or an old injury. These small problems are usually caused by latent trigger points, and over time they can snowball into more profound troubles. Other muscles may take on the job of the weakened muscle, and then *those* muscles get trigger points and may start referring pain elsewhere.

What Is Self-Care?

Our self-care protocol has four components:

1. Warming Up
2. Compression Treatment
3. Stretching, Contracting, and Relaxing
4. Movement

Many activities incorporate one or two of these concepts. For example, tai chi focuses on movement through a full range of motion, yoga focuses on stretching and strength, and fitness classes often start with a warm-up, then progress to aerobic exercise, some strengthening, and then a cooldown. For chronic muscular pain, one approach might help for a while. But the most effective way to eliminate pain is to combine all four: warming up, compression treatment, stretching, and gentle range of motion exercises. Each muscle chapter describes the first three steps in detail. You'll find all of the range of motion exercises in chapter 16.

Stage 1: Warming Up

What is warming up, and why is it important? Effective self-care treatment depends on the body being relaxed. Although warming up won't magically relax muscles containing active trigger points, it does help prevent activation of trigger points in other muscles as you treat those causing your pain.

Warming up has three components: relaxation, temperature, and blood flow. Actual warming of the body tissue is beneficial for relaxation and lengthening of muscles. A good option is taking a warm bath or shower before or even during self-care. Or you can use Fomentek hot water bags or Mother Earth Pillows to warm the area you're going to treat for 5 to 10 minutes before treatment. If you're sensitive to cold and your house is cold or drafty, use a space heater to make one room comfortable and warm, at least while you're doing self-care.

The use of heat doesn't have to be restricted to self-care. You can use hot water bags or heated pillows while traveling back and forth to work, throughout the day, or while sleeping—pretty much anytime you're sitting or lying down. This is something you can do for your muscles that doesn't take time from other activities.

A small percentage of the population (less than 2 percent) is hypersensitive to heat. If this is true of you, don't use heat as part of your warm-up or treatment.

The second component of warming up is movement, to promote circulation. This can include walking, dancing, or just standing and moving your muscles through their nonpainful range of motion before treatment. Gentle contraction and relaxation of muscles (which occurs naturally with movement) is a good warm-up and tends to promote trigger point release. If movement of any kind is painful for you, just let the application of heat and a warm room serve as the principal means of relaxing your muscles prior to compression.

Those who are sensitive to pressure or who have particularly tight muscles and fascia may find an alternative method of warming up helpful: You can actually desensitize the skin, fascia, and muscles by light brushing, a gentle salt scrub, or even self-applied massage over the areas that are tight and painful. You can do this in the shower or tub, or while lying down in preparation for treatment.

Stage 2: Compression Treatment

Compression treatment is the application of pressure on soft tissue, primarily muscles, but also other tissues, including ligaments, tendons, fascia, and skin. It can be done by hand or with various tools. If you are in severe pain, compression can also be done by friends, family members, or trained practitioners. Each muscle chapter offers treatment guidelines for practitioners at the end; those sections will also be useful for anyone wanting to assist you with compression, which can be particularly helpful in early stages of treatment.

Ways to Apply Self-Compression

Each muscle chapter includes illustrations of the muscle, its referred pain pattern, and where to look for trigger points. You can apply compression with your elbow, thumb, finger, knuckle, or self-care tools, including Backnobbers, Jacknobbers, balls of varying diameters and hardness, foam rollers, and even warm pillows. (Chapter 3 describes all these tools in detail.)

When we treat patients in our clinic, we prefer to use our elbows, thumbs, fingers, or knuckles for compression because this allows us to sense changes in tissue that we wouldn't be able to feel if we were using tools. However, when you treat yourself it's different. It will probably be better for you to use self-care tools for a few reasons: First, while you're using a tool you'll be able to feel changes in the tissue directly because you're treating your own muscles. And second, there are many areas that may require treatment (especially for low back pain) that you won't be able to reach with your hands or elbows. So in general, use your hands or elbows to treat muscles you can easily reach, such as the soleus or the abs, as long as this isn't tiring or difficult for you. Otherwise, use the most effective tool for the particular location and the condition being treated.

Chapter 3 is devoted solely to self-care tools. You'll have better results from self-care if you use these tools to assist you. We include detailed instructions for compression of specific muscles in the muscle chapters.

How Much Compression Is Enough?

The simplest answer to the question of how much pressure to use is "just enough." By that, we mean to your level of tolerable discomfort. In our clinic, we use the standard subjective pain scale from 0 (pain free) to 10 (unbearable pain). This scale is used by many physicians and practitioners when treating muscular pain. During treatment, we ask people to tell us when we're getting near a level of 6 out of 10. This should be a level of moderate, tolerable, manageable discomfort—a level that doesn't cause you anxiety. We also use the term "hurting good," meaning that the sensation of pain is often accompanied by a feeling of "that's it," or "I know that's where my pain is coming from."

You'll know you're using too much pressure if you begin to tighten up all over or feel upset. If this happens, or if you exceed a pain level of 6 out of 10, back off by applying less pressure, distributing your weight somewhere else, or modifying your compression position. It's very important that the rest of your body stay relaxed during compression treatment. Over time, as your dysfunctional muscles improve, the same level of pressure will cause less pain. As this happens, you can increase the pressure gradually until you reach the same pain level of 6 out of 10.

The Importance of Gradual Compression

Always apply and release compression gradually. Start off gently, and gradually increase pressure to the point of tolerable discomfort as you exhale. If you don't feel hardness or pain as you compress an area, slowly release the compression over about 4 seconds, then move on to the next area to be treated (as described in the muscle chapters and indicated by the X's on the muscle illustrations) and resume compression. When you press into a spot and feel resistance, hardness, or pain, either in and around the spot you're pressing or in the area where this muscle refers pain, you've located a trigger point.

When compressing a trigger point, hold the pressure for at least 10 seconds, as long as you don't exceed a pain level of 6 out of 10. As you feel the pain subsiding and are able to relax, you can increase the pressure gradually during any single application—again, just as long as you don't exceed a pain level of 6 out of 10. It's alright to prolong the compression for as much as 20 or even 30 seconds, if you remain relaxed and continue to breathe slowly and normally. It works best to increase compression slowly while exhaling.

You can take as little as 5 seconds to release pressure on a given spot; just be sure to release gradually. The benefit of compression doesn't depend on a precise duration, but rather on the application and release being done gradually, coordinated with breathing when possible, and held to a point of tolerable discomfort but not beyond. You want to perform compression in a way that maximizes relaxation of the entire body. You'll know you're doing it correctly if you feel a little less pain and more ability to lengthen and shorten the muscles you've just treated. You'll know you're doing it incorrectly if you tense up all over, if you feel worse afterward, or if bruises develop.

What Tools Do I Need?

The choice of self-care tool depends on how far along you are in the process of recovery. You should choose the tool that best helps you achieve the level of compression you can comfortably tolerate on any given day. Over time, you'll want to use more advanced types of compression, as described in each muscle chapter.

For example, when you first begin treating your gluteal muscles, you may be able to tolerate only the mildest pressure, such as a folded warm Mother Earth Pillow beneath your buttocks. Two weeks later, you may be able to easily withstand the pressure of a somewhat soft inflatable ball placed between your buttock and the wall. Then, as your muscle dysfunction decreases, you might apply compression on the floor with that same ball further inflated to make it firmer. And finally, after perhaps a month of daily self-care, you may be able to use an even harder ball on the floor while stretching the gluteals at the same time. As you can see from this example of how self-care changes over time, you might end up using three or four different tools over a period of a month to treat the same muscle.

Where Do I Apply Compression?

The MYO compression illustrations in each muscle chapter and in the appendix show you where to apply compression treatment. Look for the X's in these muscle pictures. The circled X's are the most likely places to find trigger points. Nevertheless, you should apply compression to the entire length of the muscle, shown by the smaller X's. In fact, trigger points can also occur at the attachments and tendons, so it's best to apply compression to the entire muscle. If you have trigger points in a particular location, it will feel exquisitely sensitive when you compress them and may even send referred pain to other muscles. This tells you you're on the right spot. This is valuable information and part of the reason why we say it "hurts good." Remain relaxed and continue to apply compression to this area until you feel the pain decrease. Then continue on with the rest of your self-care routine.

In most cases, you'll want to treat the same muscle on both sides of the body, even if you have trigger points on only one side. The torso muscles that are mirror images of each other often work together doing the same job, and within this relationship they're referred to as *synergists*. When a muscle has trigger points, its synergist often develops them as well, sometimes due to overworking to compensate for the muscle that first developed trigger points.

Stage 3: Stretching, Contracting, and Relaxing

Stretching is good, but combining it with contraction and relaxation is much better. *Stretching* is a gradual lengthening of muscle tissue while taking the beginning and ending of the muscle (*origin* and *insertion*) as far apart as possible. However, if you have trigger points and taut bands in a muscle, you generally won't be able to achieve full shortening or lengthening of the muscle.

How Do I Stretch?

The most important guideline for stretching is to start with the gentlest and least painful approach and gradually increase the extent and duration of the stretch as you feel the muscle gaining in flexibility. You can stretch actively or passively, by using gravity, by shortening the opposer muscles, or by first contracting the muscle and then lengthening it.

Using the abdominal muscles as an example, you can do a very gentle passive stretch by simply lying flat on your back in bed and gradually raising your arms over your head. When you can do this without pain, you can add to the stretch (passively) by placing a small pillow under your back, providing a greater arch when you lift your arms over your head. You can further increase the stretch (again passively) by allowing one leg to fall off the side of the bed. If this is too painful at first, you can place a chair next to the bed and rest your foot on it to limit the extent of the stretch.

It also helps to vary the direction of a stretch over time to target different muscle segments. Suppose you're stretching your gluteal muscles while lying face-up on the floor. As you use your arms to pull your left knee toward your chest the first time, pull it toward the center of your chest. On the second stretch, pull it halfway between the center of your chest and your right armpit. The third time, pull your knee toward your left armpit. In this way, you're actually giving a good stretch to different muscle fibers in the gluteus maximus.

Anytime you're stretching while lying down or seated on the floor, a carpeted surface is preferable. If a suitable carpeted area isn't available, use a yoga mat.

How Do I Contract and Relax?

Stretching interspersed with contraction and relaxation is always more effective than just stretching alone. This is because tight and dysfunctional muscles will be more relaxed after a mild contraction against resistance. So once you've brought a muscle to its maximum pain-free stretch and held that position for anything from 10 to 20 seconds, or a couple of slow, relaxed breaths, next move in a way that will shorten, or contract, the muscle. This involves using the muscle in the direction opposite the stretch, against resistance using about 30 percent of your strength. In most cases you don't actually move, you just push against resistance, holding the contraction of the muscle for at least 15 seconds. Then allow the muscle to completely relax as you exhale before repeating the stretch once again, stretching a little bit farther if possible. With all sequences of stretching, contracting, and relaxing, use longer intervals at first followed by progressively shorter intervals.

For example, let's say you're lying face-up on your bed and pull your thigh toward your chest to stretch your gluteus maximus. If you then press your leg away from your chest while holding it immobile with your hands (resistance), this contracts the muscle. Maintain this contraction for at least 15 seconds, then coordinate your exhalation with a complete relaxation of all effort. Then repeat the process, pulling your thigh a little closer to your chest, and stretching it for 10 seconds, and then repeat one more time, stretching for 5 seconds. It's usually possible to achieve a slightly greater stretch each time by alternating stretching and resistance. A series of three repetitions of the entire sequence is recommended, and should be followed by taking the muscle through its full range of motion a few times.

Stage 4: Movement

Movement sounds simple, but most of us get too little of it during the average day. Without adequate movement, our muscles eventually become shortened and tight. They develop trigger points and stop performing their normal functions. This is when pain sets in.

You may feel that you move all day, and wonder if that counts. It does count, but it usually isn't enough. We have a special meaning for the word "movement" in the context of our four-stage self-care protocol. In self-care, movement means taking a muscle through its full nonpainful range of motion, and doing it repeatedly to help restore full healthy range of motion to a muscle that has developed a more restricted range.

Even the most sedentary of us walk at least a modest distance every day. Casual walking doesn't qualify as a range of motion exercise, but if you walk in a deliberate way to stretch and contract the muscles of your legs and buttocks, you can take that daily walking and turn it into a useful exercise that will help restore range of motion to many of those same muscles. This can be as simple as walking a few minutes a day with your toes pointed inward and then outward. This will give a gentle stretch and contraction to several buttock and thigh muscles. This can be done anytime during the day as you walk around your home or office.

Movement is usually done actively, but it can also be done passively. *Passive movement*, which requires no effort, is movement assisted by another person, or by gravity. An example of passive movement might be another person raising your leg as you lie on your back. *Active movement* is nonstressful movement initiated by you, such as lifting your leg yourself. Chapter 16, Range of Motion Exercises, includes a variety of movements that can be used as a component of self-care treatment for all muscles that cause low back and buttocks pain. To keep things simple, we've arranged the exercises in protocols, one for each muscle covered in the book (with the gluteus maximus, gluteus medius, and gluteus minimus covered by one combined protocol).

How Often Do I Perform Self-Care?

Performing several shorter self-care sessions throughout the day works better than one long marathon session. Two 15-minute sessions a day will be enough for some people. But if your pain is severe, three, four, or even more short sessions a day may be necessary for the first few weeks, or until the pain becomes more manageable. This may require some changes in your life. You may need to get up a few minutes earlier in the morning. You may need to do self-care at work. If you're a fitness enthusiast, you may need to pause during your routine to do self-care, and you may need to do self-care immediately after your workout. However, once you become familiar with your self-care, it can even be done while watching TV. And even if it does take time or require changes, remember, this kind of self-care is the key to getting control over your pain and reclaiming your life.

Should I Change My Self-Care Program Over Time?

You need to modify your self-care program continually, a little bit at a time. Your first goal is simply to reduce the severity of your pain. The key to this is to do your initial self-care program gently and often. You may need to repeat your self-care as many as four times daily at first. That may sound like a lot, but each self-care session may take only 10 minutes. As the pain abates, you can reduce the frequency of treatment, but you should also consider increasing the duration of treatment through repetition, as well as gradually increasing the intensity.

If you spend most of each day in one position, it's especially important to do some daily self-care targeting areas that are continually used, are kept in a shortened position, or tend to feel a bit achy or uncomfortable after being in one position for too long. Our days are pretty physically active, and we do self-care every day, sometimes even every hour. For most people, one 20-minute session of self-care a day is a good investment in preventive maintenance, even after becoming pain free.

What If I Get Rid of My Pain and It Comes Back?

In every muscle chapter, we list aggravating factors that can cause trigger points in that muscle. If you get rid of your pain and it comes back, first review these aggravating factors to see if any are present. For example, high heels can often cause trigger points in the soleus or hamstring muscles, and carrying a wallet in your hip pocket can aggravate the gluteal muscles. Next, review chapter 17 to see whether any of the perpetuating factors discussed there may be a factor in your pain. Lastly, consider how consistent you've been about following your self-care routine every day. Maybe you began to let it slide a bit when the pain eased?

If you're living with chronic pain, keep noticing your pain as you continue your self-care treatment. See how your pain responds to self-treatment, and then adjust your approach as needed. It's important that you develop this skill or seek help from a practitioner who has it. If you choose the latter, you may be able to find local resources through our website, www.myopain.com.

For Practitioners

In the muscle chapters, we provide detailed explanations of various techniques for eliminating trigger points. In addition, the material in the first half of this chapter is crucial for practitioners, so please read it carefully.

Here are a few additional pointers on general techniques: Always apply compression gradually and release it gradually. Start off gently, and gradually increase the pressure as the patient exhales. Hold the pressure for as little as 6 seconds or as long as 30 seconds, making sure the patient's pain level doesn't exceed 6 out of 10. If the patient tells you the pain is subsiding somewhat, you can increase the pressure gradually as long as you don't exceed a pain level of 6 out of 10. You want to perform compression in a way that maximizes relaxation of the entire body.

When we teach our seminars, we always remind our students to compress and release in a slow, deliberate manner. This kind of treatment for the release of myofascial trigger points has always made sense to us. Here is a biomechanical explanation of the importance of performing slow compression from personal correspondence with Dr. David Simons (December 2009): "The titin molecule positions the myosin molecule and does so throughout its attachment to the z-disk. However, it must continuously exert a springlike force on the myosin and does so by folding up at its z-disk attachment. The molecule is sticky where it folds up, and getting it to unfold so the sarcomere resumes mid-range length is a slow process that is optimized by persistent gentle tension on the muscle. This is basically cytoskeletal mechanics." Dr. Simons himself tells us it is important to maintain a persistent gentle tension on the muscle. This also is a good support for our insistence on having the patient in the most stretched, supported, yet still pain-free positions for treatment.

You'll know you're doing compression correctly if the person has less pain and more ability to move the muscle through a healthy range of motion after it's been treated. During compression, make note of any referred pain created by the compression. This is valuable information that confirms the presence of taut bands of muscle with trigger points. Gliding strokes using creams or oils can also be used prior to and after compression, especially when the patient has a severely painful condition. After this trigger point pressure release, the area should be brought to further pain-free stretch, then through three full cycles of active range of motion.

Trigger Point Therapy in a Clinical Setting

In our clinic, the goal is to use myofascial trigger point therapy to help patients obtain full pain-free range of motion and full function. When people come to us, they have a specific problem and a specific outcome in mind. They have pain, weakness, or dysfunction, and they want it fixed. Our full protocol includes treatment as well as education and self-care training for the muscles that contribute to the person's problem. This is an active treatment. The patient is not a passive recipient, but rather a moving, learning, stretching participant in the journey to becoming pain free.

First we take a full history and have the person fill out a symptom or pain chart indicating where the pain is. We listen to the person's pain complaints and note the dysfunctions caused by the muscle problems. This can provide clues as to what may be causing or perpetuating the person's pain problems. Believe us: Having a practitioner listen to them is often a very novel experience for patients. They'll greatly appreciate your taking the time to listen, and more importantly, the information you gather will be crucial for effective evaluation and treatment.

As part of this initial evaluation, we assess range of motion deficits, screen for perpetuating factors, and document our findings. Then we use our myofascial referred pain charts to determine the muscles most likely to be causing the referred pain. Finally, keeping in mind the patient's goals, we develop a treatment and self-care training plan.

Behind the Techniques There's a Method

Of course, you'll need to master a set of techniques to relieve active trigger points. But behind these techniques lies a principle or method that informs everything else we do. This method is a simple feedback loop: Treat the muscles, notice the changes or improvements in the muscles, adjust the treatment, notice the changes, adjust the treatment, and so on.

This method is dynamic, continually adapting to the body's response. After all, no book can tell you exactly what to do to eliminate pain, because each pain is unique. To optimize your effectiveness, you must learn a *process* we've developed over many years. If we can pass it on to you, you'll be able to relieve other people's pain (and your own, if that's an issue), and you'll realize that every single pain problem is another lesson in how to do it. Developing an awareness of subtle changes will help you continue to adapt treatment as needed. And over time, you'll get better at it.

When we train new therapists, we teach them to think about treatment in two ways: normalizing dysfunctional tissue, and feeling the muscle's response. In this way we are actually evaluating the condition of the tissue and treating it at the same time. Every compression, stretch, movement, and contraction leaves the muscle tissue a little more or less painful, more or less flexible, or more or less strong.

A Key to Successful Treatment: Positioning During Compression

Trigger point compression can be performed while the patient is in many different treatment positions, including neutral, on the stretch, and during active or passive range of motion.

No matter what position you choose, the comfort of the patient should be your primary concern. We generally try to find the most stretched position the patient can tolerate, because treatment is most effective in a stretched position.

Treatment in the Neutral Position

Neutral position means a natural resting position with the muscle being treated neither shortened nor lengthened. We usually begin the first treatment in this position because it places the least stress on the patient, who doesn't yet know you and may not trust you. This position also allows you to determine the person's baseline sensitivity to compression. For example, you can compress a prone patient's paraspinals and ask them to tell you how much discomfort the compression causes on a scale of 0 to 10. You can then adjust the compression to find the level you're looking for: 6 out of 10.

Treatment on the Stretch

Each muscle chapter includes numerous examples of how to treat the muscle in its stretched position. This position is beneficial for a variety of reasons:

- Quite often, the taut bands will actually stick out, making them easier to find.

- Compression is often less painful.

- Taut bands are more likely to release under compression.

- You accomplish two things at once: treating the trigger points and retraining the muscle by extending it to its normal stretched length.

- When you treat the taut bands and they release, the stretch will usually increase, providing confirmation that the treatment is working.

Treatment After Contracting the Muscle

It's critical for the patient to be actively engaged in treatment. We always instruct the patient to use and move the muscles in various positions, often against slight resistance that we provide. This promotes blood flow to the tight areas and helps retrain the muscles and restore their full function. To this end, we recommend you incorporate contraction movement as part of treatment. For example, while treating the hamstrings with the patient lying prone, you can resist at the heel while the patient tries to bring the knee into further flexion by contracting the hamstrings. Hold this for 10 seconds, then have the patient relax. Feel for changes in the hamstring muscles and surrounding tissue. See if the taut bands are more relaxed or if the painful spots are less painful. You can then treat any spots still containing trigger points.

During active contraction and passive movement, consider these questions: Is the patient able to actively extend or internally or externally rotate the muscle or muscles? What muscles are primarily employed for the given motion? Does the person have any pain during movement? If so, where is it? Does the muscle contract when it should be relaxed, such as during passive shortening or lengthening? Does it feel as though one muscle or segment of muscle feels bigger or denser on one side than the other? The answers to these questions can help you develop an effective treatment plan.

Clear signs of myofascial dysfunction include pain with movement or compression (or even just being touched), twitching of the muscles, inability to completely relax after muscular effort, or any inhibition of normal movement. With the hamstrings, it's especially common to find some or all of these problems. You and your patient can measure progress as you demonstrate greater range of motion during compression or less twitching or pain during movement or compression.

Treatment During Passive Range of Motion

When you find a taut band containing trigger points, you can treat it while moving the part of the body being treated. As the trigger points release, you'll notice an increase in the muscle's range of motion. This immediate feedback confirms that the treatment is working. As an example, when you treat the hamstring muscles with the patient prone, move the lower leg back and forth and up and down. As the hamstring trigger points release, you should notice a greater range of pain-free movement.

Treatment During Active Range of Motion

Treatment while the patient is actively moving the muscle through its range of motion is another very effective treatment technique. An example would be treating the paraspinal muscles with the patient in a seated position and flexed forward to stretch the paraspinal muscles. Have the patient slowly extend the stretch more, and also bend to the right and left. Notice whether there is pain or restriction during any of these movements, then see if the range of pain-free movement increases after treatment of the areas containing trigger points.

Stretch Range of Motion

As you'll read throughout this book, one way to check for the presence of trigger points in specific muscles is to measure any deficits in their stretch range of motion. However, it's important to bear in mind that several muscles may play a role in achieving that stretched position. So you may deduce from a supine knee to chest test that the patient has trigger points in their gluteus maximus, yet after treatment the person still can't pass the test. In this case, it's important to check to see what the iliopsoas and abdominals are doing when passively shortened, as they need to be fully relaxed to pass the test. If these muscles contain active trigger points, they may involuntarily contract.

Muscles can have dysfunction in all positions. For our purposes, *passive shortening* is when a practitioner moves the muscle into a shortened position without any effort being exerted by the patient or the muscle itself. If the muscle tightens in this position, it can be caused by taut bands and active or latent trigger points within the muscle. There can also be chronic passive shortening; for instance, in the iliopsoas and abdominal muscles from sleeping all night scrunched up in a fetal position. In such a case, when the person stands up straight or tries to extend the hip, they experience muscle pain and trigger point activation.

Heat and Cold

If you follow sports, surely you're aware that ice is the most commonly mentioned treatment for sports injuries. You can't go a day without reading about some athlete being iced down. The general idea is that this somehow reduces or prevents pain and is beneficial to healing. This is, at best, a misunderstanding. Ice has two primary effects: It deadens the sensation of pain, and it reduces swelling after an injury. But cold treatment can also shorten muscle fibers and activate trigger points, making an athlete more susceptible to injury while performing.

For most people, unless they're in almost unbearable pain, heat is more helpful. It can be easily applied before, during, or after treatment. As part of our clinical therapy, we sometimes sandwich the patient between hot water bags, warm flaxseed pillows (microwaveable), or hydrocollator packs. Heat relaxes the muscles. It also relaxes the person in general. In addition, heat sends a sensation message to the central nervous system that temporarily replaces the pain messages from trigger points. Cold can also provide distraction from the pain sensation and is best used while stretching the taut bands containing trigger points, as we do with the spray and stretch technique described below.

Spray and Stretch

Spray and stretch is another technique that can help restore full pain-free range of motion to dysfunctional muscles. The spray part of this technique refers to thin, cold streams of vapocoolant sprayed in parallel sweeps onto the skin over active trigger points and over the area of referred pain caused by these trigger points. When applied with the patient in a stretched position, it will almost immediately eliminate even very severe pain or reduce it very markedly. The vapocoolants we generally use are Instant Ice (available over the counter) or Spray and Stretch (available only to licensed professionals).

The stretch part of the technique refers to the fact that while the practitioner is spraying the coolant, the muscle being sprayed is simultaneously stretched a bit farther while the patient remains relaxed and comfortable. This stretching of taut bands in the muscles promotes circulation to the muscle and surrounding fascia and is a wonderful relief for muscles that have been restricted.

Patient Self-Care

After treatment, the patient should be encouraged to follow a self-care program as described in this book. It's important to explain that this can play a significant role in the person's rehabilitation. Although you can relieve some pain for many patients who refuse to do self-care, it takes longer and they're more likely to experience a relapse when treatment ends.

Chapter 3

Useful Self-Care Tools

If you want to get rid of your pain and keep it from recurring, you need to make a modest investment in self-care tools. We've used these products for many years, and we've found them well adapted to the self-care needs of our patients. They're well made, and the manufacturers stand behind them. Considering the countless thousands of dollars many of our patients have squandered on tests and failed treatments before they ever found their way to our doors, the cost of these tools is trivial and a very good investment in your recovery.

We recommend some products by brand name. These products are not the only ones on the market, and you may find others that work as well. Some of the recommended products are available through our website (www.myopain.com).

You can do a lot with your own hands and a few things you can find around the house (tennis balls, baseballs, volleyballs, beach balls, a dog leash, and heating pads). Especially in an emergency or if you're simply strapped at the moment, we're in favor of using what's on hand for immediate relief.

But if your goal is not only to correct the most severe problems causing your pain, but also to condition your muscles so you won't face that pain again, spending a few hundred dollars on self-care tools could be the best investment you ever make. Think about your car for a moment: If you have front end problems or you need new brakes, you spend the money to have it done and done right. That kind of repair could easily run to a thousand dollars or more—and for routine maintenance, the bill won't be covered by insurance. If you're willing to spend that kind of money to keep your car safe and reliable, don't shy away from spending a small fraction of that on keeping yourself free of pain and fully functional. These tools are durable, and even when used daily, they'll help you for a very long time before you'll ever need to replace them.

Another good reason to have self-care tools on hand is that you can stress or overuse your hands and arms while trying to achieve the compression needed for treating trigger points. And when treating low back and buttocks pain, there are quite a few places you can't easily reach with your own hands. In these cases, self-care tools will provide you with the leverage and pressure you need.

You need to learn where and how to use these tools. In the individual muscle chapters, we tell you where to use them. In this chapter, we provide more detail on when, why, and how to use them. The tools we recommend can be divided into four categories:

- Compression tools

- Conditioning tools

- Sources of heat or cold

- Other treatment aids

Compression Tools

Different compression tools are appropriate in different contexts. For example, some are more appropriate for treating certain muscles. Or you may choose a tool depending on the tenderness or size of the area being treated. In addition, sometimes it may be worthwhile to combine tools, for example, using a strap to facilitate stretching while using another tool to provide compression. All the treatment techniques mentioned below are described in detail and illustrated in the muscle chapters.

Backnobber

The Backnobber (see next page, figure 3.1) could be considered the forefather of trigger point self-care tools. The first product designed by the Pressure Positive Company, it was created specifically for treatment of trigger points back in the late 1970s. We've used it for over twenty-five years and have never had a problem with the product or the company that makes it.

The Backnobber is a curved S-shaped tool designed to easily reach the neck, shoulders, back, and buttock areas. There are two kinds of Backnobbers: The Original Backnobber is a one-piece metal S-shaped hook with wooden knobs at each end that apply the pressure. The Backnobber II is made of fiberglass reinforced nylon and can be separated into two smaller pieces for easy storage and portability.

The Original Backnobber comes in three sizes. The Big Bend version is especially useful for taller or larger people. This tool is able to reach around the torso or waist of a larger person and can be used to easily compress any of the muscles in the back and buttocks.

Because the Backnobber II separates into two smaller pieces, it's a better choice if you travel a lot. Whenever we travel somewhere, we take along a Backnobber II. It's easy to use half of it to treat the muscles at the base of the skull and neck, and the entire S-shaped tool for other areas.

Backnobbers can be used just about anywhere but are intended to be used over lightweight, dry clothing. Using the tool after a soak in the hot tub or after a hot shower or bath will enhance trigger point release by combining the therapeutic effects of the warm or hot water with the compression applied by the tool. When using these tools, keep your hands relaxed; don't squeeze or grip the tool tightly. Let's say you have trigger points in your paraspinal muscles. You can compress those trigger points very easily using the Backnobber by slipping one end beneath your back while lying face-up on a carpeted surface. Press gently outward and down on the other end as shown in figure 3.1, to achieve just the amount of pressure you want.

The advantage of the Backnobber for treating back and hip muscles is that you can easily move the tool from one area to another while keeping your body in a fixed position. With most of the other compression tools we discuss below, you'll need to move your body over a tool (a ball or a Jacknobber) that remains in the same place. This can require a bit of coordination and muscle strength, and if you're in a lot of pain to begin with, that can be stressful.

That's where the Backnobber is the ideal choice for self-care.

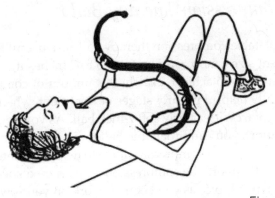

Figure 3.1

Jacknobber

The Jacknobber (see figure 6.13 on p. 82) is a small tool that resembles a large version of the jacks you might have played with as a child. The multidirectional prongs allow the tool to be stabilized on the floor or against a wall, chair back, or seat bottom while you press your muscles into it. The prongs also make it possible to maintain the tool in a proper alignment to achieve compression while lying, sitting, or leaning into it. The four prongs are of slightly different size so you can adjust the amount of compression on a particular spot by choosing a different prong. There are variations on this product from different companies, made of plastic, wood, or wood and metal. Pressure Positive offers a variety of differently shaped tools that all accomplish the same basic function: compression from a small hand tool. These tools include the Jacknobber, the Index Knobber, and the Knobble. We prefer the Jacknobber for treating muscles in the back, gluteal muscles, hips, hamstrings, quadratus lumborum, and soleus, especially while sitting.

Tennis Balls and Other Balls

You may have tennis balls around the house. Actually any ball will do, but we particularly like the texture and relative hardness of a tennis ball. It's easily managed by putting it into a knee-high (or full-length) stocking so you can control it while working with it. You do this by holding one end of the stocking while throwing the other end (containing the ball) over your shoulder and pressing your lower back or hips into the ball against a wall. The tennis ball is the cheapest self-care tool. It's also versatile, easy to pack, and easy to use. Because of its small size, a tennis ball may give you a little too much compression at first. So try it, and if you experience too much discomfort, choose a larger or softer ball, or other self-care tools altogether. But once you're no longer in acute pain, a tennis ball or a racquetball, which is somewhat firmer, is probably the easiest choice for compression because you can use it anywhere you can find a wall to lean against or a chair to sit on.

Compression Therapy Balls

Inflatable compression therapy balls are useful for compressing larger areas. They come in several different sizes, most ranging from 5 to 7 inches in diameter. Because they're inflatable, you can adjust the hardness to achieve exactly the amount of compression you want or can tolerate. These balls are especially helpful in early stages of treatment, when areas with active trigger points may still be very tender. Start with a fairly soft 7-inch ball. As you begin to deactivate trigger points and experience less discomfort, you can inflate the ball more to make it harder, use a smaller ball, or both. A harder ball will apply greater compressive force to help stimulate circulation to the muscles and fascia. The smaller the ball, the more the compression focuses on a specific area. A 7-inch diameter ball is more versatile and a better choice as you begin to work on your own muscle problems.

At the very beginning, you can use this ball while lying in bed. If the bed is soft, you won't feel a great deal of compression from the ball even if it's pretty firm. As your muscles become less sensitive to the compressive force, you can try rolling against the ball on a wall with the ball against your gluteal muscles, paraspinals, or abs. As you progress further, try using the ball on the floor. Sometimes a compression therapy ball that feels just right against the wall may feel too firm for use on the floor, so you may need to deflate it slightly.

When using a compression therapy ball on the floor, be sure to maintain control of your body as you roll on and off the ball. If necessary, hold on to a sofa or large chair to help you control your rolling movements. When rolling on a compression therapy ball, wear gym shoes so you'll have enough traction to control your movement. Also, it's best to roll on the ball on a carpeted or padded surface. A yoga mat works well if you have only hard wood or tile floors. You can purchase compression therapy balls at our website (www.myopain.com).

Foam Rollers

We use several different kinds of foam rollers—thicker, thinner, softer, harder—depending on individual needs. Probably the most versatile is a 3-foot-long roller with a 4-inch diameter and a hard PVC core. You can easily find smaller foam rollers sold as "pool noodles," and also larger rollers with a 6-inch diameter. You might consider getting one of each size, but if you can afford only one, get the roller with a 4-inch diameter.

A roller is most easily used on the floor by pressing your body weight onto it as you roll slowly over it. The foam roller gives broader, more diffuse pressure than the various "knobber" tools, and it's more stable than balls of almost any size. This makes the foam roller a better choice when you're at an early stage of treatment or need to treat a larger area (such as the entire back) in a short time. You can use it quickly to treat the back, abdomen, buttocks, thighs, and lower legs.

Orbit Massager

The Orbit Massager, made by the Pressure Positive Company, can be used to provide smooth, diffused compression to areas that are particularly painful. Since it has a strap that goes around the user's hand, it need not be gripped and therefore doesn't fatigue the hand.

Conditioning Tools

Conditioning tools are items that aid in retraining muscles for full, dynamic function. Among the wide variety available, we feel that fitness balls and dynamic movement disks are the best. Using these items stimulates the muscles to work without excessive fatigue or stress.

Fitness Balls

Larger-diameter fitness balls can be obtained almost anywhere. Many companies offer conditioning or fitness balls ranging from 45 to 65 centimeters in diameter. These large balls are used primarily for stretching and conditioning the postural (core) muscles. When using the ball for conditioning, you sit on the ball, either on a small fixed circular base that prevents it from rolling out from under you or, if you're in good shape, simply on the floor without a base. Unless you're in exceptional condition, you'll need to work up to being able to sit on these balls with good posture for even 5 minutes. The idea is to move slightly from side to side and back and forth on the ball to stretch and strengthen the core muscles of the torso, particularly the paraspinals, which help stabilize and control movements of the spine. It's not a good idea to use these large balls when you're still in an acute phase of trigger point activation and pain. Wait until you are in much less pain before trying them.

Dynamic Seating Disks

These disks perform in much the same way as fitness balls but can be transported easily, can be used on top of any chair, and can be inflated or deflated to accommodate the level of dynamic seating you can tolerate. Dynamic seating means the surface you're sitting on isn't hard and fixed; it's fluid and requires your core muscles to work to keep you stable. Don't overdo it at first. Start by sitting on the cushion no more than 5 minutes out of every hour, and gradually work up to 15 minutes per hour. These cushions can be used as dynamic standing devices also, in which case the cushion should be minimally inflated so it will be more stable. As you gain confidence and balance, you can inflate it a bit more fully.

Stretching Straps

Stretching straps are an effective tool for gradually increasing stretched range of motion safely. We recommend the 6-foot Stretch Out strap, which contains stitched loops at 6-inch intervals so you can easily adjust the amount of stretch applied. It's important to remain relaxed when using this tool. Don't squeeze or grip the loops any harder than necessary to maintain control. The many stitched loops make it easy to see your progress; as you become more flexible, you'll be able to move to new positions on the strap. These straps are inexpensive, well made, and better adapted for stretching the legs and hips than a dog leash (which is an option if you don't have a strap). You can also make a stretching strap from clothesline.

Sources of Heat and Cold

When muscles hurt or are chronically tight, it can be very relaxing and soothing to place heat over the area. It can also be empowering to do something very simple to reduce your pain. And as mentioned in chapter 2, pressure, cold, skin brushing, and heat are all effective ways to break the cycle of pain, tightness, and more pain. Any source of heat is useful as a broad sensation distraction. When the body is distracted by the sensation of heat, it isn't so focused on the referred pain caused by trigger points. This allows you to apply compression without feeling as much pain. Once you feel the warming, you can begin to treat the area.

Mother Earth Flaxseed Pillows

Mother Earth Designs makes a variety of pillows filled with flaxseeds that retain heat for a considerable time. We've used these pillows for over ten years. They can be purchased either scented or unscented. We like them because after they're microwaved for a few minutes, they retain heat for up to half an hour, so they can be easily used before, during, or after treatment. Microwaving time depends on the size of the pillow; just be careful not to overdo it. We start with 1 minute and add more heat in 1-minute intervals as needed. To distribute the heat more evenly through the pillow, take it out of the microwave after 1 minute, move the flaxseeds around, and then microwave for another minute, repeating as needed.

Mother Earth Pillows are a useful heat source that can help you relax anytime, and they can be very useful when you're in acute pain or experiencing spasms. We use these pillows primarily as a warm-up for the muscles prior to compression, stretching, and range of motion exercises. We also use them after treatment to relax the patient, and sometimes use them as the gentlest form of compression when a patient is in extreme pain.

There are several different shapes and sizes of Mother Earth Pillows. The large flat pillow is probably the most useful for heating the entire lower back and buttocks regions. Microwave it to reach a tolerably high level of heat (as warm as you can stand against your skin without discomfort). If it becomes too hot, just wrap it in a towel. This pillow is a bit heavy and is best used at home.

Small flat flax pillows are versatile, lighter, and a good choice for traveling or everyday use at home, at work, in the car, in a hotel, and so forth. These smaller pillows provide heat over an area of roughly 6 by 10 inches.

The Shoulder Trigger Point Pillow can be used in place of a traditional doughnut-shaped coccyx cushion for sitting. This pillow is also good for heating the quadratus lumborum area and the abdominal obliques, because you can wrap it around your waist, back, or buttocks.

The Mother Earth Body Wrap is about 24 inches long by 4 inches wide. It's useful for applying heat and gentle compression on the spine from the tailbone to the mid-thoracic region. It can also be wrapped around the waist just above the buttocks.

Fomentek Bags

Fomentek bags can be filled with either hot or cold water to apply heat or cold. They're easy to use and are much more flexible than the traditional hot water bottle your grandmother may have given you when you were suffering with aches and pains. Simply fill them between one-fourth and one-third full with warm water, then squeeze down on the bag to "burp out" all the air before sealing. Place the cap on firmly, until it snaps, then wipe off the outside of the bag if it got wet during filling.

We generally prefer heat for muscle relaxation and recommend using water as hot as you can tolerate without discomfort. You can also use cold water to help with acute pain or spasm. The advantage of Fomentek bags is that they conform to your body. You can place one underneath your back while lying in bed and it will stay warm for up to an hour. It's best to use these bags inside a pillowcase or wrapped in a towel, or while wearing light clothing, so they don't lie directly against your skin.

Fomentek water bags come in three sizes: large, small, and mini. The large size (18 by 24 inches) is very good for warming a large area but may be too heavy for some people when filled. The small size (15 by 18 inches) is very manageable and still large enough to heat the entire buttocks or low back region. The mini (11 by 15 inches) bag is lightweight and handy. Another great use of these bags is to provide a dynamic seating surface. This permits small movements of the pelvis so that you aren't stuck in a fixed position for a long time while sitting.

Instant Ice

Instant Ice is an aerosol vapocoolant spray that can be purchased directly by the consumer. A vapocoolant spray allows you to temporarily desensitize severely painful areas so you can restore some flexibility to dysfunctional muscle tissue that you couldn't otherwise treat or stretch. Use of this product is described in detail in the "For Practitioners" section of chapter 2. It serves as a mild surface anesthetic, giving you temporary relief from referred pain and allowing you the chance to begin self-care treatment in situations where you would otherwise feel in too much pain to try anything.

Other Treatment Aids

There are a few other tools you might find useful, such as skin brushes and massage creams or oils. And because poor seated posture and ill-fitting chairs play such a major role in low back pain, you might also want to invest in a seat wedge. It's also important that chairs and other furniture fit your body well, and that your workspaces have good ergonomic design. We'll discuss this more specifically in the muscle chapters.

Brushes

If you are in a lot of pain, using a soft bath brush can be a good form of treatment to start with. It serves as a distraction from pain and, used gently, is soothing and tends to help reduce sensitivity in the underlying muscles, at least for a short time. It can be especially effective if done in a hot bath or shower. This also helps muscles relax and lengthen. Brush over the muscles containing trigger points as well as the entire area of referred pain.

Oils and Creams

If you're sore after compression, massage the muscles containing trigger points and the areas of referred pain, using long, gliding strokes. Using cream or oil is helpful. Only massage muscles you can reach without straining, such as your abdomen, hamstrings, or soleus, and keep in mind that it's best to stretch the muscles as you massage them.

Angled Footrests and Seat Wedges

While technically not self-care tools, angled footrests and seat wedges provide postural support and can help those with chronic muscle problems caused or exacerbated by too much sitting. Angled footrests help push your back into the back of the chair and prevent your hamstrings from pressing into the front edge of the chair. In a pinch, a book on the floor can be used for this purpose; place your heels on the front edge and angle your toes to the floor.

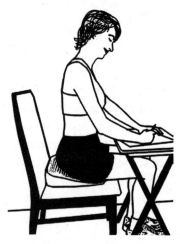

Figure 3.2

While it's best to have a well-designed chair that's completely adjustable (height, seat angle, armrest height, and back angle), you can accomplish a lot with a simple seat wedge. The seat wedge prevents you from assuming poor seated posture, also known as *kyphosis*. Using a seat wedge angled toward the front of the chair promotes good seated posture with proper lumbar curvature, as shown in figure 3.2. Seat wedges are made from different materials, including soft foam, harder foam covered with vinyl, and memory foam. Some are inflatable, which has the advantage of allowing you to move your pelvis forward and back and side to side. Even slight pelvic movements every few minutes can help prevent trigger points from developing. Also, you can inflate or deflate the wedge to provide exactly the support you need to give you an ideal lumbar curve.

For Practitioners

We highly recommend you become familiar with the tools in this chapter and use them on yourself so you can recommend them to patients. Most patients want to take responsibility for their recovery, and motivated, empowered patients will be your best ally in obtaining a successful treatment outcome. Plus, if you're a hands-on therapist, low back pain and hand and arm pain are the two most common afflictions you personally will face over your career. These are also two of the most common reasons people leave the field. So for hands-on therapists, the first benefit of learning to use self-care tools is career longevity. In addition, they're fun and really make a difference in the health of your muscles. By using them yourself, you can recommend them based on your own personal experience and can better train your patients in the self-care protocols in this book. Both you and your patients will benefit from this proactive approach to therapy. Motivated patients who have these tools and the knowledge to use them will be a great credit to your abilities, even if they end up doing most of the work!

Testing Tools

A *pressure algometer* measures the amount of pressure (usually in pounds per square inch) that can be applied at the limit of a patient's tolerance. For example, a patient with a severely contracted soleus muscle came to us a few years ago and initially couldn't tolerate pressure greater than 2 pounds. After two weeks of treatment, she was able to comfortably stand pressure above 15 pounds. The pressure algometer objectively demonstrated the progress after myofascial trigger point therapy.

A *goniometer* can be used to measure the angle of any given joint at maximum stretch. For example, it can measure the angle at the hip joint when a person stretches forward toward their toes while seated on the floor. Objective measurements can help document changes in response to treatment, and the findings can be useful when communicating with other health care providers, for research, or to clearly document findings if needed for insurance reimbursement.

Algometers can cost more than five hundred dollars, and goniometers cost around twenty dollars. Both are most useful for practitioners who work regularly with chronic pain.

Body Support Systems

Body support cushions can significantly improve the effectiveness of myofascial trigger point therapy. They allow you to treat the patient in a stretched position while maintaining good support. And in many positions, the support system takes pressure off the side or area the patient is lying on. This can make a huge difference if an area was previously too painful to lie on. You can find more information about body support systems on our website: www.myopain.com.

Tools or Hands?

Don't think of the self-care compression tools described earlier in the chapter as substitutes for your hands. Your hands remain the best tools for treating your patients. This is because the hands are a two-way mechanism for any skilled practitioner. In addition to providing treatment, sensitive hands can detect the presence or absence of taut bands of muscle tissue, as well as changes in tissue during treatment. So your thumbs, fingers, knuckles, and elbows are the best tools to use when treating anyone other than yourself.

One Final Note

In the treatment sections of several of the muscle chapters, we offer the option of treating the patient through a warm Fomentek bag. If you do this, it's best to place the bag inside a pillow case so the bag is not applied directly against the patient's skin.

Chapter 4

Index of Low Back Pain Symptoms

This chapter can serve as a "cheat sheet" for those of you anxious to get to your goal—pain relief—as soon as possible. It includes two resources: images of common pain referral patterns for the muscles covered in this book, and an extensive table of symptoms, keyed to the muscles that may harbor trigger points responsible for those symptoms.

The easiest approach is to review the following illustrations of pain referral patterns. If any of these images resembles your pain pattern, turn to the chapter for that muscle to learn how to do self-care for the muscle. The muscle chapters also include other helpful information, such as causes and perpetuating factors for trigger points in that muscle.

Pages 43, 44, 45, 46, 47

These illustrations by Barbara D. Cummings are used with kind permission from Dr. David G. Simons, from the book he coauthored with Dr. Janet Travell, *Myofasical Pain and Dysfunction: The Trigger Point Manuals Volumes I and II*

Iliopsoas pain referral patterns (see chapter 5)

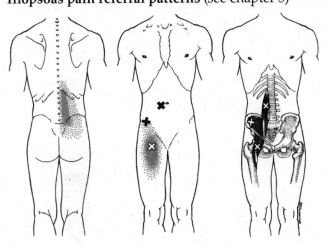

Paraspinals pain referral patterns (see chapter 6)

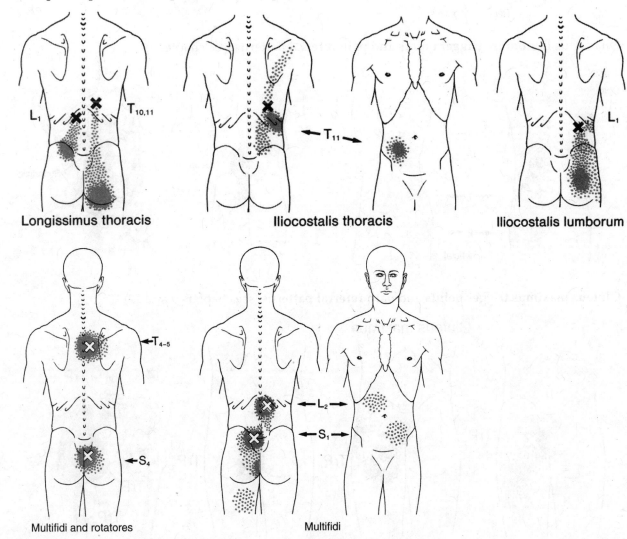

Longissimus thoracis

Iliocostalis thoracis

Iliocostalis lumborum

Multifidi and rotatores

Multifidi

Rectus abdominis trigger points and pain referral patterns (see chapter 7)

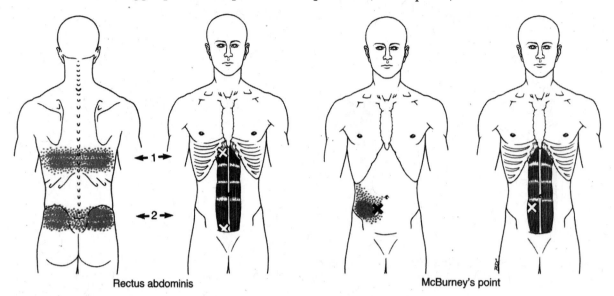

Rectus abdominis   McBurney's point

Quadratus lumborum trigger points and pain referral patterns (see chapter 8)

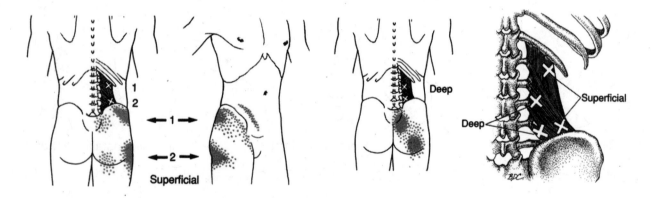

Gluteus maximus trigger points and pain referral patterns (see chapters 9 and 12)

Gluteus maximus

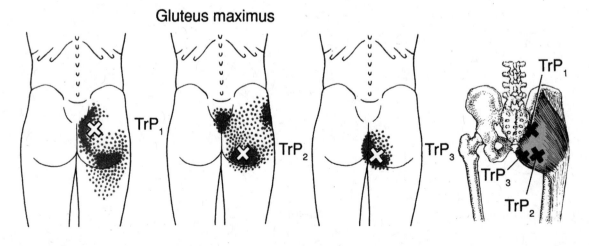

Gluteus medius trigger points and pain referral patterns (see chapters 10 and 12)

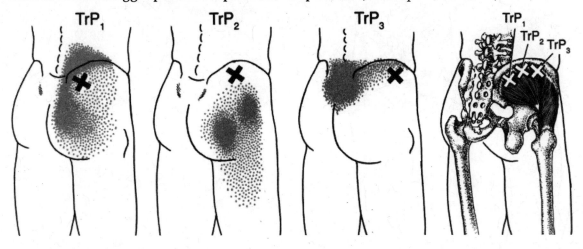

Gluteus minimus trigger points and pain referral patterns (see chapters 10 and 12)

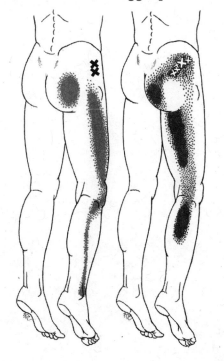

Piriformis trigger points and pain referral patterns (see chapters 11 and 12)

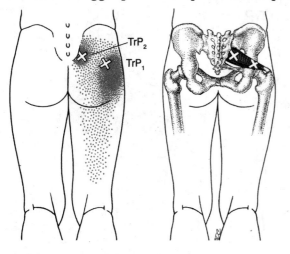

Hamstrings trigger points and pain referral patterns (see chapter 13)

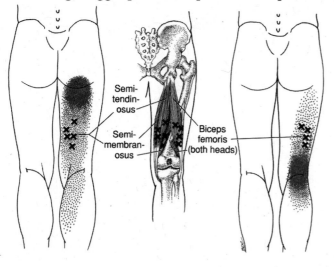

Soleus trigger points and pain referral patterns (see chapter 14)

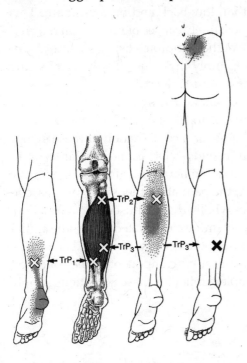

Another approach is to consult the table on the following pages, in which we've compiled a list of symptoms that may indicate the presence of trigger points responsible for pain in the low back and buttocks. These symptoms include a variety of different kinds of pain and dysfunction. The relevant symptoms are also listed and described in detail in each of the muscle chapters in the sections entitled "Do I Have Trigger Points in My…?"

Using this table is pretty straightforward. Just scan the left-hand and center columns of symptoms, which describe different kinds or locations of pain and things you may have difficulty doing or that cause pain when you do them. Look for the symptoms that describe your problem, then look across to the right-hand column for the muscle or muscles most likely to cause that pain or dysfunction. To be a little more precise, what you'll find is the muscles most likely to contain trigger points causing that pain or dysfunction. There is considerable overlap; some symptoms indicate possible trigger points in two, three, or more muscles. Even so, in many cases that helps you narrow down the list of suspect muscles. Where more than one muscle is listed, they're listed in the order in which they are likely to harbor trigger points causing the symptom in question.

After locating your symptoms, go to the relevant chapter or chapters and start reading. Each muscle chapter offers a number of ways to confirm or rule out trigger points in that particular muscle. If you determine that the first muscle doesn't contain trigger points, you can go on to the next suspect muscle. If you're not sure, there's a foolproof way to figure out whether a muscle contains trigger points: Just treat it, stretch it, and move it. If your pain or other symptoms diminish noticeably or go away, you've found the problem.

When using this table, keep in mind that other muscles not covered in this book could be causing or contributing to the pain, particularly for symptoms other than low back and buttocks pain. This table lists only the muscles covered in this book, which are the most likely causes of myofascial referred pain in the low back and buttocks. Also, keep in mind that some of the symptoms listed, such as incontinence, often have nonmuscular causes. The muscles listed are simply those most likely to cause the dysfunction if the cause is muscular and related to your low back or buttocks pain.

Important note: A number of diagnostic terms are included among the symptoms listed in this chapter, including paresthesia, sciatica, radiculopathy, osteoarthritis, and scoliosis. These are all conditions associated with low back pain, numbness, tingling, weakness, or a combination of these symptoms. Some practitioners may also refer to pseudo-radiculopathy, pseudo-sciatica, and similar terms in recognition that there can be causes for these symptoms other than the nerve impairment or arthritic condition usually deemed responsible for the symptoms. In fact, the pain and other symptoms associated with these conditions can often be partially or in some cases wholly due to muscular dysfunction. Unfortunately, the muscular component of such pain is rarely examined or treated. Once the initial diagnosis is made, the book is often closed. We list these diagnoses here because if you've been given one of these diagnoses, it's worthwhile to consider the possible muscular component of the condition or ask your physician to do so. You may find partial or even complete relief for these conditions simply by evaluating and treating the myofascial symptoms.

General Location or Problem	More Specific Area or Problem	See Muscle Chapter
Abdomen	Pain in the upper or middle abdomen	Rectus Abdominis, 7 Paraspinals (deep), 6
	Pain in the lower abdomen	Rectus Abdominis, 7 Quadratus Lumborum, 8 Paraspinals, 6 Pelvic Floor Muscles, 15
	Cramping in the abdomen	Rectus Abdominis, 7
	Sagging abdominal muscles	Rectus Abdominis, 7
Achilles tendonitis and pseudo-Achilles tendonitis	Posterior ankle and heel pain	Soleus, 14
Ankles	Limited range of motion	Soleus, 14
	Swelling	Soleus, 14
Asymmetry, standing	Postural asymmetry	Iliopsoas, 5 Quadratus Lumborum, 8 Paraspinals, 6 Rectus Abdominis, 7 Gluteus Medius, 10 Gluteus Minimus, 10 (also see chapter 17)
Back pain	Pain across the low back	Rectus Abdominis, 7
	Pain up and down next to the spine	Iliopsoas, 5 Paraspinals, 6
	Severe aching "bone pain" at any level of the spine	Paraspinals (deep), 6
	Can't hold back straight, slouched-forward posture (kyphosis)	Paraspinals, 6 Iliopsoas, 5 Rectus Abdominis, 7 Gluteus Medius, 10 Gluteus Minimus, 10
Breathing	Increased back pain with deep breathing	Rectus Abdominis, 7 Paraspinals, 6
	Paradoxical breathing (contracting the abdominal muscles during normal inhaling)	Rectus Abdominis, 7 (also see Psychological Factors, in chapter 17)

General Location or Problem	More Specific Area or Problem	See Muscle Chapter
Buttocks	Any pain in the buttocks	Quadratus Lumborum, 8 Gluteus Maximus, 9 Gluteus Medius, 10 Gluteus Minimus, 10 Piriformis, 11 Paraspinals, 6 Hamstrings, 13 Soleus, 14 Pelvic Floor Muscles, 15
	Pain that extends to the lower leg and calf	Gluteus Minimus, 10
	Pain in the center of the buttocks and around the sacrum	Gluteus Medius, 10 Gluteus Maximus, 9 Piriformis, 11
	Aching deep in the buttocks	Gluteus Maximus, 9 Paraspinals, 6 Quadratus Lumborum, 8 Gluteus Medius, 10 Piriformis, 11 Rectus Abdominis, 7 Soleus, 14 Pelvic Floor Muscles, 15
Car or chair	Difficulty getting in or out of a car or chair	Iliopsoas, 5 Rectus Abdominis, 7 Paraspinals, 6 Gluteus Minimus, 10 Gluteus Maximus, 9 Quadratus Lumborum, 8 Hamstrings, 13
	Can't seem to find a comfortable seated position	Gluteus Maximus, 9
Coughing	Extreme pain while coughing	Quadratus Lumborum, 8 Rectus Abdominis, 7

General Location or Problem	More Specific Area or Problem	See Muscle Chapter
Feet	Swelling	Soleus, 14
	Turning out of feet (laterally rotating at hip)	Gluteus Medius, 10 Gluteus Minimus, 10 Gluteus Maximus, 9 Iliopsoas, 5 Hamstrings, 13 (also see Morton's Foot Syndrome in 17)
Gastrointestinal disorders	Heartburn, nausea, vomiting, loss of appetite, bloating, indigestion, burning, swelling, and gas	Rectus Abdominis, 7
Groin	Pain	Quadratus Lumborum, 8 Rectus Abdominis, 7 Pelvic Floor Muscles, 15 Iliopsoas, 5
Growing pains	In children's legs	Soleus, 14 Hamstrings, 13
Heels	Pain, soreness, or aching at night	Soleus, 14
Hips	Pain that totally immobilizes the hips	Quadratus Lumborum, 8
	Bursitis and pseudo-bursitis, severe pain or tenderness in and around the hip bone (the greater trochanter of the femur)	Quadratus Lumborum, 8 Gluteus Minimus, 10
	Limited ability to flex the hips	Iliopsoas, 5 Gluteus Maximus, 9 Gluteus Medius, 10 Gluteus Minimus, 10
	Pain or inability to move thigh or leg backward (hip extension)	Gluteus Maximus, 9 Hamstrings, 13 Iliopsoas, 5 Quadratus Lumborum, 8 Paraspinals, 6 Gluteus Minimus, 10 Gluteus Medius, 10
	Weakness in the hips	Gluteus Medius, 10 Gluteus Minimus, 10
Irritable bowel syndrome	Constipation, abdominal pain, or diarrhea	Rectus Abdominis, 7
Knees	Pain in the back of the knee	Hamstrings, 13

General Location or Problem	More Specific Area or Problem	See Muscle Chapter
Legs	Difficulty lifting a leg out to the side (hip abduction)	Gluteus Maximus, 9 Gluteus Medius, 10 Gluteus Minimus, 10 Piriformis, 11
	Leg length inequality	Iliopsoas, 5 Quadratus Lumborum, 8 Gluteus Medius, 10 Gluteus Minimus, 10 (also see chapter 17)
	Limping	Gluteus Minimus, 10 Gluteus Medius, 10 Soleus, 14 Hamstrings, 13 (also see Leg Length Inequality in chapter 17)
	Restless legs syndrome (involuntary twitching of leg muscles, especially at night or while lying down)	Iliopsoas, 5 Gluteal Muscles, 9 & 10 Hamstrings, 13 Paraspinals, 6 Soleus, 14
	Tingling in the legs and thighs	Piriformis, 11
	Tingling in the thighs only	Iliopsoas, 5
	Pain in the buttocks and down the thigh and leg (sciatica)	Gluteus Minimus, 10 Hamstrings, 13 Piriformis, 11
Lordosis	Excessive low back or lumbar curve (anterior tilt of pelvis)	Iliopsoas, 5 Paraspinals, 6 Quadratus Lumborum, 8 Gluteus Medius, 10 Gluteus Minimus, 10

General Location or Problem	More Specific Area or Problem	See Muscle Chapter
Low back (lumbar region)	Generalized pain in the lumbar region	Iliopsoas, 5 Rectus Abdominis, 7 Paraspinals, 6 Gluteal Muscles, 9 & 10
	Lumbago (an older term for very low back pain in and around the sacrum)	Gluteus Medius, 10 Gluteus Maximus, 9 Paraspinals, 6 Quadratus Lumborum, 8
	Sharp pains that may make it impossible to stand or walk	Quadratus Lumborum, 8 Paraspinals, 6 Iliopsoas, 5 Rectus Abdominis, 7
	Pain running across the low or mid back	Rectus Abdominis, 7
	Pain running up and down the low back parallel to the spine	Iliopsoas, 5
	Pseudo-osteoarthritis of lumbar or sacral regions of spine	Paraspinals, 6 Quadratus Lumborum, 8 Iliopsoas, 5 Rectus Abdominis, 7 Gluteal Muscles, 9 & 10 Piriformis, 11 Soleus, 14 (also see Small Hemipelvis in chapter 17)
Lying down	Pain while lying down or sleeping, barely able to turn over	Quadratus Lumborum, 8 Gluteus Minimus, 10
	Buttocks pain after long bed rest with legs always bent	Hamstrings, 13
	Pain when sleeping on your side	Gluteus Medius, 10 Gluteus Maximus, 9 Gluteus Minimus, 10 Piriformis, 11 Quadratus Lumborum, 8 Hamstrings, 13
	Pain from lying on your back with your legs straight	Gluteus Maximus, 9 Piriformis, 11

General Location or Problem	More Specific Area or Problem	See Muscle Chapter
Menstrual pain	Severe cramping	Rectus Abdominis, 7 Paraspinals, 6
Nausea *(see Gastrointestinal disorders)*		
Numbness, tingling, or heightened sensitivity (paresthesia or hyperesthesia), by area	Ankle or foot	Piriformis, 11 Soleus, 14
	Buttocks, hips, perineum	Gluteus Maximus, 9 Piriformis, 11
	Groin, scrotum, or labia	Iliopsoas, 5 Piriformis, 11
	Legs	Piriformis, 11
	Low back	Piriformis, 11
	Front of thighs	Iliopsoas, 5
	Back of thighs	Piriformis, 11 Hamstrings, 13
	Spinal region, skin over and around	Paraspinals, 6
Postural asymmetry *(see Asymmetry, standing)*		
Radiculopathy and pseudo-radiculopathy	Numbness, tingling, or weakness in various muscles, thought to be due to nerve root problems but often caused by muscular dysfunction	Paraspinals, 6 Quadratus Lumborum, 8 Iliopsoas, 5 Rectus Abdominis, 7 Gluteal Muscles, 9 & 10 Piriformis, 11 Hamstrings, 13 Soleus, 14
Rectum	Pain	Pelvic Floor Muscles, 15
Restless legs syndrome *(see Legs: Restless legs syndrome)*		
Sacroiliac joint	Pain in or around	Paraspinals, 6 Gluteus Maximus, 9 Gluteus Medius, 10 Quadratus Lumborum, 8 Rectus Abdominis, 7 Piriformis, 11 Soleus, 14 Pelvic Floor Muscles, 15
	Stabbing pain in or around the joint, or in the lower buttocks, abdomen, hips, or groin	Quadratus Lumborum, 8

General Location or Problem	More Specific Area or Problem	See Muscle Chapter
Sciatica or pseudo-sciatica	Pain in the buttocks and down the side and back of the thigh or down the outside and back of the lower leg	Gluteal Muscles, 9 & 10 Hamstrings, 13 Piriformis, 11 Iliopsoas, 5 Paraspinals, 6 Quadratus Lumborum, 8 Soleus, 14
Scrotum (including the testes)	Pain	Iliopsoas, 5 Quadratus Lumborum, 8 Piriformis, 11
Sexual dysfunction	Painful intercourse	Piriformis, 11 Pelvic Floor Muscles, 15 Rectus Abdominis, 7
	Impotence	Piriformis, 11
Sitting	Pain from prolonged sitting	Gluteus Maximus, 9 Iliopsoas, 5 Rectus Abdominis, 7 Piriformis, 11 Hamstrings, 13 Quadratus Lumborum, 8 Pelvic Floor Muscles, 15
	Pain when getting up from a sitting position	Iliopsoas, 5 Paraspinals, 6 Gluteus Maximus, 9 Piriformis, 11
Sleeping (*see Lying down*)		
Slouching	When seated, with back rounded forward	Rectus Abdominis, 7 Paraspinals, 6
Sneezing	Extreme pain when sneezing	Quadratus Lumborum, 8 Rectus Abdominis, 7

General Location or Problem	More Specific Area or Problem	See Muscle Chapter
Spine (*also see Torso, bending*)	Abnormal curvature (scoliosis and functional scoliosis)	Quadratus Lumborum, 8 Iliopsoas, 5 Paraspinals, 6 Rectus Abdominis, 7 (also see Mechanical Factors in chapter 17)
	Deep aching pain on one or both sides of the spine	Paraspinals, 6
	Pain with any movement of the spine	Paraspinals, 6
	Severe "bone pain" in any part of the spine	Paraspinals, 6
	Sharp pains along the spine	Paraspinals, 6
Squatting	Heels don't touch floor when squatting	Soleus, 14
Stairs	Back and buttocks pain when climbing stairs	Iliopsoas, 5 Quadratus Lumborum, 8 Gluteus Maximus, 9 Hamstrings, 13 Paraspinals, 6 Soleus, 14
	Restricted range of motion while climbing stairs	Gluteus Maximus, 9 Gluteus Minimus, 10 Gluteus Medius, 10 Iliopsoas, 5

General Location or Problem	More Specific Area or Problem	See Muscle Chapter
Standing	Heel pain while standing	Soleus, 14
	Pain when standing	Quadratus Lumborum, 8 Iliopsoas, 5 Rectus Abdominis, 7 Paraspinals, 6 Piriformis, 11 Soleus, 14
	Severe pain when standing upright	Quadratus Lumborum, 8 Gluteus Minimus, 10
	Slouching while standing	Rectus Abdominis, 7 Iliopsoas, 5 Paraspinals, 6 Quadratus Lumborum, 8 Hamstrings, 13
	Difficulty standing on one leg	Gluteus Medius, 10 Gluteus Minimus, 10 Quadratus Lumborum, 8 Soleus, 14
	Always standing with feet turned out (lateral rotation at hip)	Gluteal Muscles, 9 & 10 Iliopsoas, 5 (also see Morton's Foot Syndrome in chapter 17)
Swelling	Of the feet and ankles	Soleus, 14
Swimming	Low back pain while swimming	Paraspinals, 6
	Difficulty or weakness doing the flutter kick (hip extension)	Gluteus Maximus, 9 Hamstrings, 13 Paraspinals, 6
Tailbone (coccyx)	Deep pain around the tailbone	Gluteus Maximus, 9 Pelvic Floor Muscles, 15 Paraspinals, 6
Thighs	Pain, numbness, tingling, or heightened sensation in the front of the thigh	Iliopsoas, 5
	Pain, numbness, tingling, or heightened sensation in the back of the thighs	Hamstrings, 13 Gluteus Minimus, 10 Piriformis, 11
	Pain in the inner thighs	Pelvic Floor Muscles, 15

General Location or Problem	More Specific Area or Problem	See Muscle Chapter
Toes	Difficulty in touching the toes	Hamstrings, 13 Soleus, 14 Gluteus Maximus, 9 Paraspinals, 6 Iliopsoas, 5
	Difficulty pushing off the toes while walking or running	Soleus, 14 Gluteus Medius, 10 Gluteus Minimus, 10 Quadratus Lumborum, 8
Torso, bending	Sharp pain upon bending forward and to the side that seems to come out of nowhere	Quadratus Lumborum, 8 Paraspinals, 6 Iliopsoas, 5 Rectus Abdominis, 7 Gluteus Maximus, 9
	Pain while arching backward	Paraspinals, 6 Quadratus Lumborum, 8
	Pain while bending forward	Paraspinals, 6 Quadratus Lumborum, 8 Iliopsoas, 5 Rectus Abdominis, 7
	Difficulty or pain bending or leaning to either side	Quadratus Lumborum, 8 Paraspinals, 6 Rectus Abdominis, 7
Urination	Frequent urination or occasional incontinence	Pelvic Floor Muscles, 15 Rectus Abdominis, 7
	Bladder spasm	Rectus Abdominis, 7
Vagina	Pain, intense burning	Pelvic Floor Muscles, 15
	Deep soreness after intercourse	Pelvic Floor Muscles, 15 Hamstrings, 13
Vertebrae	Severe aching "bone pain" in the spine	Paraspinals (deep), 6 Rectus Abdominis, 7 Iliopsoas, 5

General Location or Problem	More Specific Area or Problem	See Muscle Chapter
Walking	Abnormal limping gait	Gluteus Medius, 10 Gluteus Minimus, 10 Piriformis, 11 Hamstrings, 13 Soleus, 14
	Unbearable pain when walking	Quadratus Lumborum, 8 Soleus, 14
	Pain in general when walking	Gluteus Medius, 10 Gluteus Minimus, 10 Quadratus Lumborum, 8 Pelvic Floor Muscles, 15 Hamstrings, 13 Soleus, 14
	Can't walk on tiptoes, or difficulty walking up or down hills or stairs	Soleus, 14
	Back pain while walking uphill, especially with the torso flexed forward	Gluteus Maximus, 9
	Difficulty shifting weight from side to side while walking	Soleus, 14 Gluteus Medius, 10 Gluteus Minimus, 10 Quadratus Lumborum, 8
	Shortened stride	Soleus, 14 Hamstrings, 13 Iliopsoas, 5 Gluteus Medius, 10 Gluteus Minimus, 10 (also see Morton's Foot Syndrome in chapter 17)
	Weakness in the hips when walking	Gluteus Medius, 10 Gluteus Minimus, 10 Piriformis, 11 (also see Morton's Foot Syndrome in chapter 17)
	Buttocks pain when walking uphill	Soleus, 14
	Difficulty walking with knees bent	Soleus, 14
	Heel pain when walking	Soleus, 14

Chapter 5

Iliopsoas

In our experience, trigger points in the iliopsoas (pronounced IL-e-o-SO-as) cause more low back pain than those in any other muscle. This is especially noteworthy when you consider that many people haven't heard of the iliopsoas, and some muscle charts don't even show it. Trigger points in the iliopsoas are a problem in more than half of our low back pain cases. Many times, correcting problems in the iliopsoas completely eliminates the pain. Because of its location, when the iliopsoas is involved, eliminating pain in the back requires treatment from the front of the abdomen.

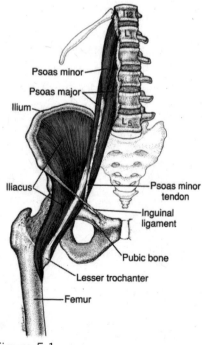

Figure 5.1

Where Are the Iliopsoas Muscles and What Do They Do?

The iliopsoas includes two muscles—the psoas and the iliacus—both attaching at their lower end to the inside of the thighbone just below the pelvic region, as shown in figure 5.1. The longer of the two, the psoas, lies deep within the abdominal cavity and attaches to the front of the lower vertebrae. It runs down and forward through the lower abdomen to the inside edge of the femur a few inches below the hip socket. The iliacus attaches to the entire inner surface of the large, fan-shaped pelvic bone and runs down inside the pelvis, where it merges with the psoas proper. There are, of course, right and left iliopsoas muscles, and it's possible to have trigger points in one or both sides.

The iliopsoas muscles are almost constantly at work, as they help stabilize the upper body and keep the torso erect whenever we're sitting or standing. The density of these muscles diminishes with age, and because the psoas is important in lifting the leg when running, this may explain why running at top speed gets harder as we get older. These muscle frequently perform other tasks, as well:

- Because they help us bend at the hip and lift the thighs toward the chest, they're always active when walking, jogging, running, or climbing stairs.

- They assist in pulling the legs together and turning the leg out.

- They do a lot of the work involved in sit-ups if the feet are stabilized in one position.

Iliopsoas Pain Referral Patterns

The iliopsoas contains three primary trigger point regions that all can cause pain that runs up and down the low back parallel to the spine, as shown in the left-hand image in figure 5.2. The uppermost trigger point region is inside the abdomen near the spine, about two inches to either side of your belly button. Since it is deep in the abdomen, you will need to press through the relaxed abdominal muscles straight into the abdomen toward the spine. You can also treat this area with compression by start-ing outward of the belly button four inches, then pressing downward and on an angle toward the spine.

The middle trigger point region is inside the ilium. Locate your iliac crest and move down along it about one inch. Move inside the rim and press back into the ilium. The third and lowest trigger point in the iliopsoas is in the upper thigh. Active trigger points in this area cause pain in the front of the thigh and also into the low back (Travell and Simons 1992).

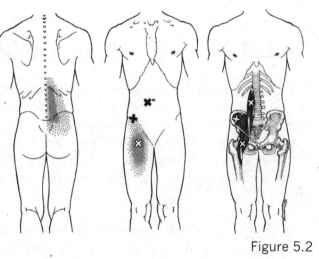

Figure 5.2

What Aggravates the Iliopsoas?

A number of activities can cause or exacerbate taut bands in the iliopsoas:

- Too much time in a seated position (the most common aggravating factor)

- Sudden overloading of the muscle, such as catching yourself when slipping on ice

- Driving for long periods or driving in a low seat with your knees higher than your buttocks

...ng in a fetal position, which shortens the iliopsoas, or sleeping on your stomach, ...h stretches the iliopsoas (see chapter 17 for more on sleep positions)

...mbar spinal surgery

...coliosis

- Using your leg to move a heavy object, or repetitive kicking, as in karate or soccer

- Long bike rides in a bent-over position

- Holding chronic abdominal tension

Of all these aggravating factors, by far the most important is the first: too much sitting. Unfortunately, it can be difficult to avoid this, and we have to admit that we're sitting now as we write this book! We sit as we drive back and forth to work. We sit at mealtimes. We sit during meetings, while watching TV and movies. In short, many people sit much of the day, and far more than they should. Since many of us can't just stop sitting, the key is to break it up with self-care treatments, stretching, and range of motion exercise, which can help offset the ill effects.

Do I Have Trigger Points in My Iliopsoas?

Pain running up and down the low back parallel to the spine is the most reliable indicator of trigger points in the iliopsoas. However, when both right and left iliopsoas muscles are contracted, you might also feel pain running across your low back. With either pain pattern, it's reasonable to suspect the iliopsoas is involved and needs attention. You can find out for sure by treating the muscle. If the pain diminishes or goes away completely, you have (or had) trigger points in the iliopsoas.

In addition to these pain patterns, several other problems point to the iliopsoas as the main culprit:

- When you stand, you are slightly bent forward at the hip (with or without pain) or tend to bend forward and twist to one side, indicating that one side of the iliopsoas is contracted.

- You have difficulty rising from a seated position.

- You experience back pain whenever you try to stand completely straight.

- You have difficulty getting out of a low couch or a car seat.

- The pain can be so severe that you may be reduced to crawling on your hands and knees.

Simple Tests

Two simple tests can help you determine whether your iliopsoas has trigger points: the seated chest to thighs test and the straight leg raise and hold test.

Seated Chest to Thighs

This test determines whether your iliopsoas can shorten normally. Sit in an upright chair with a firm seat, bend forward at the waist, and allow your chest to rest on your thighs as shown in figure 5.3. If you're able to bring your chest down to your thighs with no pain in either your thighs or your low back, your iliopsoas is functioning normally. If you can't bring your chest down to your thighs or if you experience pain in your low back, you have trigger points in your iliopsoas, or possibly in the muscles in your back that you're stretching.

If you carry extra tummy weight, that may restrict your ability to fully bend your torso forward and down onto your thighs. In that case, it's more important to notice any feelings of tightness in the iliopsoas muscle itself (in your abdomen) or pain in your low back as you assume this bent-forward position. If you don't experience any pain or tightness during this test, your iliopsoas muscles are probably okay.

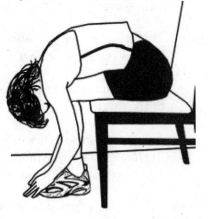

Figure 5.3

Straight Leg Raise and Hold Test

This test was developed by Dr. Hans Kraus, one of the pioneers in the field of physical fitness and myofascial trigger point therapy. He called it the minimum fitness test for the posture muscles. **Caution:** Do not attempt this test if you've been diagnosed with bulging disks.

Lie face-up flat on the floor. Tilt your pelvis up and press your low back into the floor. If possible, have a partner check to see that your lower back is flat on the floor. Keep both legs straight and raise them a foot above the floor, as shown in figure 5.4. Hold this position for 10 seconds while keeping your low back flat against the floor. If you're able to keep your legs up while holding your back flat against the floor, you don't experience low back pain, and your muscles aren't quivering, your iliopsoas muscles are okay and have the minimum strength needed to maintain normal posture. If your low back comes off the floor, if you feel pain, or if you can't hold your legs up for 10 seconds, you probably have trigger points in the iliopsoas. If it's at all painful to raise your legs or hold them off the floor, put them down and consider this test a positive indicator for trigger points in the iliopsoas.

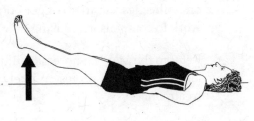
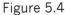

Figure 5.4

Helpful Hints for Eliminating Trigger Points in the Iliopsoas

In addition to self-care treatment, there are a few other simple things you can do to help avoid or alleviate trigger points in the iliopsoas:

- When driving for long periods, make frequent stops to stand and stretch. If you experience low back pain while driving, take stretch breaks as often as necessary to alleviate the pain—even every 20 minutes.

- Vary your sleeping position to allow for extension of your leg or torso (see chapter 17 for more on sleep positions).

- Use warm Fomentek bags or Mother Earth Pillows on your abdomen and down to the top of the thigh.

- Tip your chair seat forward slightly if it's adjustable. If it isn't, use a seat wedge, as described in chapter 3, so your thighs slope downward while sitting. Alternatively, consider buying a kneeling chair to use intermittently.

- Check your mattress to ensure that it's neither too soft nor too firm.

Self-Care Treatment

Here are a few general pointers to keep in mind for all the compression techniques and stretches described in this chapter:

- Warm the area prior to treatment, especially when your symptoms are severe.

- When sitting or lying on the floor for any form of self-care (compression, stretching, range of motion exercises), a carpeted surface is ideal; alternatively, you can use an exercise mat.

- Treat both sides, even if you appear to have trigger points on only one side. The two sides are synergists and often work together to do the same job, so trigger points often develop on both sides. Or after trigger points develop on one side, the other side may have to overwork to compensate, causing new trigger points to develop.

- Refer to the MYO compression illustration (5.5) and compress all areas indicated by X's. The larger circled X's represent likely spots for trigger points, but the entire muscle requires treatment.

- Never exceed a pain level of 6 on a scale of 0 to 10.

- When applying compression, sustain the compression for up to 30 seconds and repeat at least two or three times, or until there's a noticeable decrease in pain and increase in range of motion.

- Gradually increase the amount of compression as you feel the muscle softening and relaxing. Be aware of how the tissues respond to treatment.

- When stretching, hold the position for two to three normal breaths.

- When a stretch is repeated several times on both sides, alternate sides with each repetition.

- After treatment and stretching, do the range of motion exercises for the iliopsoas described in chapter 16.

Compression

For guidance on self-compression, look at figure 5.5. The larger circled X's represent the most likely places to find trigger points. However, because the entire length of a muscle can be dysfunctional, we recommend that you apply compression to the entire muscle, as indicated by the small X's, applying more sustained compression to any areas that are firmer or more painful.

To treat the iliopsoas, you need to press through the superficial muscles of the abdomen and upper thigh. To help relax the abdomen and allow for more effective compression, try placing either warm Fomentek bags or Mother Earth Pillows over your abdomen for several minutes before beginning compression.

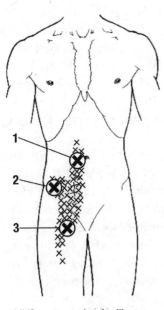

MYO compression for Iliopsoas

Figure 5.5

Beginner Level

Stand facing a wall with a 7-inch compression therapy ball placed just to the right or left of your belly button and held between your abdomen and the wall, as shown in figure 5.6. Lean into the treatment ball as you relax your abdominal muscles. If you have trigger points in the iliopsoas, this should "hurt good." Over time, as you're able to withstand greater pressure, further inflate the ball to make it firmer. The idea is to gradually increase pressure from week to week. As the muscle regains flexibility, you'll feel less discomfort during compression.

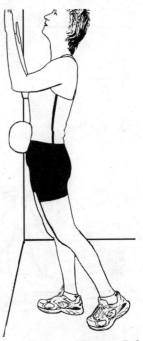

Figure 5.6

Intermediate Level

When you've achieved some improvement in range of motion of the iliopsoas, indicated by diminished low back pain and greater ease and flexibility of movement, especially when getting out of a

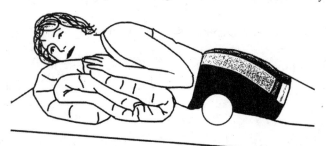

Figure 5.7

low chair or car seat, you're ready for more focused self-treatment. Lie on your side on the floor with a pillow or folded blanket under your upper body for support. Place a 7-inch compression therapy ball next to you at the level of your belly button and roll onto the ball, placing some of your body weight on the ball right over the iliopsoas, as shown in figure 5.7. Apply only as much pressure as you can easily tolerate. Hold this position for 10 seconds, then roll back onto your side again and move the ball slightly lower down your abdomen and roll onto the ball again. Continue moving the ball gradually lower until the ball is pressing into the uppermost part of your thigh.

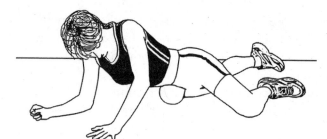

Figure 5.8

Most people begin with a softer ball and progress to a firmer ball (by inflating it) as they get more comfortable with treatment. An alternative is to progress to balls of a smaller diameter, such as a 5-inch compression therapy ball. As compression becomes less painful, try pushing yourself up on your elbows or hands, as shown in figure 5.8, so you stretch the iliopsoas as you apply compression.

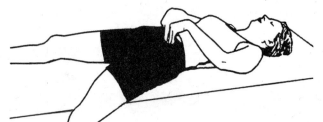

Figure 5.9

Depending on your strength and dexterity, you may achieve the same compression as with a ball by using your fingers, knuckles, or a Jacknobber. It's better to treat the iliopsoas while in a stretched position, so try treating it while lying face-up on a bed with your leg extended down, as shown in figure 5.9. Place your fingers, knuckles, or the Jacknobber about 1 or 2 inches to either side of your belly button and press in firmly for 10 seconds. Some people prefer the Backnobber because it's easy to grasp and allows you to apply more leverage, as shown in figure 5.10. In this figure, pillows are placed beneath the back to allow self-treatment while the iliopsoas is on the stretch. Compression while stretching the muscle being treated is an ideal combination—once you've restored some mobility to the muscle with gentler methods of treatment.

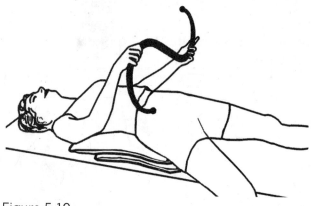

Figure 5.10

Stretching

Stretching the iliopsoas can be quite pleasurable. Often the pain abates noticeably as the muscles begin to lengthen. Several different stretches can be used alternately or in combination. In addition to the stretches below, the cobra stretch in chapter 7 (page 104, figure 7.24) is also helpful. However, it's a more advanced technique than those described here. If it causes you pain or stress, it's too soon to be doing it. You could try a modified version, doing the stretch for a shorter count, or wait until other treatments and stretches have given you greater muscle flexibility and strength.

Seated Iliopsoas Stretch

While sitting in a sturdy chair without arms, scoot over to one side of the chair and extend the leg on that same side backward while remaining in an upright seated posture, as shown in figure 5.11. Just push the leg gently down and back as far as you can. Don't worry if it won't go very far, and don't overdo it or risk a cramp. Stretch each leg at least three times and gradually extend the stretch a little farther each time.

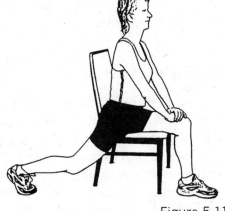

Figure 5.11

Standing Iliopsoas Stretch

For this exercise, hold on to a countertop or sturdy chair for support. Extend one leg back while maintaining an upright posture, as shown in figure 5.12. Arch your torso back a bit so your torso and leg form a curve, and try to increase the curve a little more each time you do the stretch. Stretch each leg three times. If your balance is very good, you may do this stretch with your hands by your sides, rather than holding on to anything.

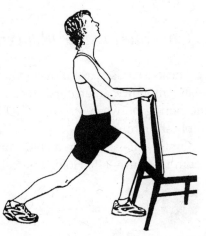

Figure 5.12

Prone Iliopsoas Stretch

Lie face-down with a thick pillow under one thigh. Lift that leg up behind you, as in figure 5.13, trying to keep the front of your pelvis and your abdomen relaxed. Do this

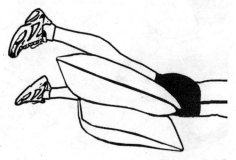

Figure 5.13

stretch three times for each leg. As you achieve greater flexibility, you can add more pillows under your thigh.

Doorjamb Stretch

Stand in a doorway and place both hands on the sides of the doorjamb above your head. With one foot forward and the other back, slowly lunge forward with your torso arched back, as shown in figure 5.14. Do this stretch three times on each side, lunging forward a little more each time.

Kneeling Stretch

To stretch the left iliopsoas, kneel on your left knee with your right foot on the floor in front of you in a lunge position. Slowly rock forward onto your right foot while gently arching your chest and torso back to provide more stretch. If you need help with balance, do this stretch in a doorway and hold on to the doorjamb. Do this

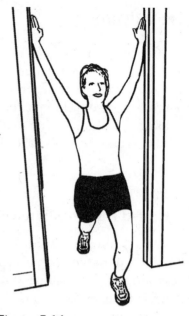

Figure 5.14

at least three times for each leg, holding for 10 seconds and striving for a little more stretch each time. Don't extend the stretch so much as to cause more than mild discomfort.

Contracting and Relaxing

These exercises use movement against resistance alternating with relaxation to help you achieve greater mobility. Intersperse these contract-and-relax exercises with the stretches described above. Alternating between stretching and contraction will give you more improvement in mobility than simple stretching alone.

First, while seated in a chair, push down on one thigh as you try to raise it at the same time, as shown in figure 5.15. Hold this resistance for 10 seconds, then exhale, relax, and stretch the leg out. Repeat three times on each side.

Another good way to help release the iliopsoas is to contract the opposing muscles, which include the gluteal muscles and the superficial paraspinal muscles. Here's one way to do that: Stand with your hands on the back of a sturdy chair. Bring one leg back and raise it about a foot off the floor as shown in figure 5.16, keeping it as straight as you can. Hold for 10 seconds, then exhale, relax, and return your leg to the floor and

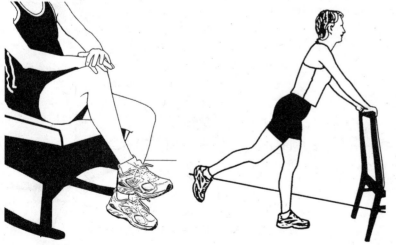

Figure 5.15   Figure 5.16

perform a standing lunge similar to the one shown above, in figure 5.12. Repeat three times for each leg, stretching your leg a bit farther back each time.

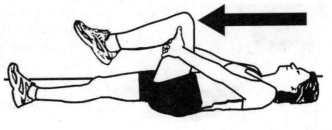

Figure 5.17

Here's another way to contract the opposing muscles: While lying face-up on the floor, bring one knee toward your chest. Hold on to the back of the thigh with your hands, as shown in figure 5.17, or if you can't reach your thigh, use a robe strap or a towel. Try to push your thigh away from you, while continuing to hold it stationary for 10 seconds. Then exhale, completely relax your abdomen, and draw your knee as close to your chest as you comfortably can. Repeat three times for each leg. As a variation, when you pull your knee in to your chest, pull it toward the opposite shoulder.

For Practitioners

It's particularly valuable for therapists to understand how to test for and treat dysfunction of the iliopsoas. Because of the muscle's location, it can be difficult for patients who are older, weaker, or suffering from severely tightened iliopsoas muscles to do self-treatment, particularly if they don't use self-care tools. You can teach these patients effective self-treatment techniques if you keep several self-care tools on hand—at a minimum, a Jacknobber and a compression therapy ball. It's also critical to help your patients restore full range of motion once you've treated and stretched the iliopsoas. Please refer to chapter 16 for a full movement program you can teach patients to do at home.

Assessment and Tests

Several simple tests can help you determine whether a patient has iliopsoas trigger points: the knee to armpit test, the Thomas test for single hip extension, and a visual test for asymmetry. Always test both sides, even if you suspect trigger points on only one side.

Knee to Armpit Test

This test checks whether the iliopsoas can shorten in a relaxed, normal manner. Have the patient lie supine with their legs straight. Bring one of the patient's knees toward and across the chest (left knee pulled over to right armpit and vice versa), and feel for any contracting when the muscle is passively shortened. Note the distance from knee to chest. If the patient can bring the knee fairly close to their chest without pain, this indicates normal (shortening) range of motion and probably no trigger points. If there is tightness in the abdomen or pelvis when the knee is brought to the chest, referred pain into the back or thigh, or the knee can't be brought within 12 inches of the chest, this indicates trigger points in the iliopsoas. However, if this occurs without pain, it could be due to extra weight in the tummy or trigger points in the gluteus maximus. It's worth noting that many top athletes have failed this test

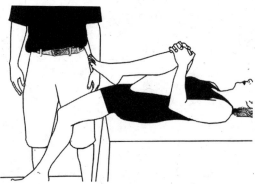

Figure 5.18

in our clinic. Muscle flexibility through the full range of motion, not just strength, is necessary for a completely functional iliopsoas muscle.

Thomas Test for Single Hip Extension

This test measures the ability of the iliopsoas to stretch normally. Seat the patient at the end of the treatment table with the edge of the table under the buttocks. Have the patient grasp one leg below the knee and draw it toward their chest. Hold the patient's upper torso (from the back) and cradle the patient as they slowly lean back onto the treatment table, keeping the straight leg relaxed. Make sure the patient doesn't slip off the table. If the thigh of the patient's straight leg is at a downward angle, as shown in figure 5.18, then the iliopsoas has no trigger points. If the extended leg is above the height of the table or if there's pain in the low back, this indicates iliopsoas trigger points.

Underlying Perpetuating Factors

Be sure to look for structural problems when you find dysfunctional iliopsoas muscles. These include a small hemipelvis, leg length inequality, and Morton's foot syndrome. (All these conditions are discussed in chapter 17.) These problems are common, yet many people go through life without being aware of them. Millions of dollars are squandered on MRIs and other diagnostic tests looking for possible causes of chronic back pain when the answer is simply structural or muscular imbalance.

Treatment Techniques

Here we'll describe some advanced techniques for restoring full pain-free function to the iliopsoas muscle. Use these after other treatment techniques, such as trigger point compression. It is most effective to use a sequence of actively contracting against resistance, holding, relaxing, and then stretching. For the first resistance maneuver, place the patient prone on the treatment table, then put your knee beneath the patient's thigh as shown in figure 5.19. Have the patient press down on your thigh for 15 to 30 seconds. Part of the benefit of this exercise is that it reduces stress on the therapist. Do this treatment at least twice on each side even if trigger points are evident only on one side.

In the next maneuver, cradle the leg in your arms while holding

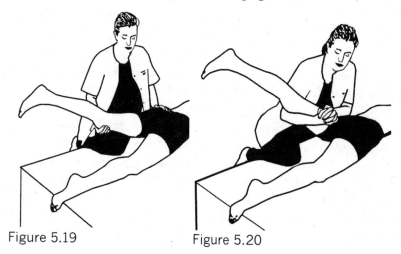

Figure 5.19   Figure 5.20

down the patient's hips with a forearm or elbow and lifting the leg to stretch the iliopsoas with the other arm, as shown in figure 5.20. Then have the patient attempt to press that thigh back to the table using 10 to 20 percent of their strength against your resistance for 15 seconds. After a coordinated exhale, have the patient fully relax while you gently lift the leg a little farther and take up the slack in the iliopsoas. With the leg slightly higher, have the patient press down again for 10 seconds with about 20 percent of their strength. Repeat this passive stretch a final time for 5 seconds. This is a very effective method for getting a chronically tightened iliopsoas to release, but it can be stressful for the therapist. Don't try this maneuver if the patient is bigger than you; it's simply too strenuous. In that case, you can place firm bolsters under the thigh for the resistance element and go through a similar procedure.

We would like to give you practitioners some general treatment suggestions for the iliopsoas. While you can certainly compress trigger point #1 through the rectus abdominis (see figure 5.5), it is also effective to first begin compression outside the lateral edge of the rectus abdominis by pressing horizontally toward the spine as you move under the rectus abdominis fibers. Specific tender areas become quickly apparent as you treat the uppermost psoas in that manner. For trigger point #2, you will need to press below the inside edge of the iliac crest and inward onto the ilium. Look for taut bands throughout the entire inside of the ilium. You can flex the patient's hip to soften the femoral portion of the iliopsoas and the abdominals. This will allow you to really reach the illiacus portion of the iliopsoas. Trigger point #3 is at the uppermost quarter of the femur, distal to the inguinal ligament and above the lesser trochanter.

Spray and Stretch

For spray and stretch, have the patient lie supine near the edge of the treatment table. Allow the leg being treated to extend off the edge of the table and gently extend the upper hip with one hand while spraying the vapocoolant over the abdomen, groin, and anterior thigh, as shown in figure 5.21. If possible, passively stretch the iliopsoas farther, add medial rotation at the hip, and spray over the abdomen, groin, and anterior thigh again. Then turn the patient onto their side and spray the lower back and buttocks in the whole area of referred pain.

Always follow spray and stretch treatment with heat to warm the skin and muscles, then have the patient move through their full range of motion for the iliopsoas three times, using the exercises in chapter 16. Finally, repeat this entire treatment on the other side. Always treat the iliopsoas bilaterally, even if most of the pain and shortening occurs on one side only. Interestingly, Dr. Travell found that although the pain caused by chronically contracted iliopsoas muscles is mostly felt in the low back, actual release of the taut bands in the muscle will respond much better to spraying on the abdomen, groin, and anterior thigh. So the effectiveness of spray and stretch depends more on treating the muscles doing the referring, as opposed to the areas where pain is felt. We like to do both front and back, in order to treat both the iliopsoas and the opposer muscles, which are often also dysfunctional.

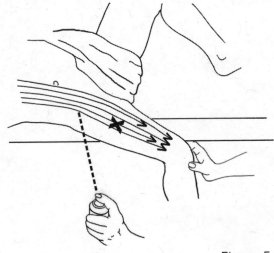

Figure 5.21

Things to Avoid

Although it's counterproductive to attempt to strengthen chronically shortened iliopsoas muscles containing trigger points, this is often what's prescribed for people who have low back pain, in the form of core strengthening exercises. However, because trigger points cause muscle weakness as well as pain, muscles that harbor trigger points will continue to be weak no matter how many core exercises are performed. Such efforts often account for a patient "failing" physical therapy. The first priority is to restore normal range of motion through compression, stretching, and the iliopsoas exercises in chapter 16. Once that has been achieved, strengthening exercises are appropriate and helpful.

Nerve Entrapment

The iliacus can entrap the femoral cutaneous nerve and cause burning and numbness in the front and side of the thigh. The iliacus can also entrap the genitofemoral nerve, causing loss of sensation in the genitals. Numbness or tingling in the genital region indicates possible trigger points in the second or third trigger point region of the iliopsoas (see figure 5.5, above). So if you detect these symptoms, you'll need to treat those two areas.

Chapter 6

Paraspinals

The paraspinal muscles include a variety of individual muscles, some very small and others quite long; some deeper and some more superficial; and some closer to the spine and some farther away. We'll use the term "paraspinals" (meaning "around the spine") to refer to all these muscles. As you look at the anatomy of this muscle group (see figures 6.1 and 6.2), you might be tempted to throw in the towel. You may think, "How will I ever find the specific muscles in my back that are causing my pain?"

The answer is that the nature and location of the pain often helps you pin it down to a pretty small area. And then there's the ultimate test of whether you've found the right muscles: If the pain diminishes or goes away entirely after you've treated the muscles, you've found the source of your pain.

Many terms associated with chronic back pain, such as herniated disks, pinched nerves, and bulging disks, seem to call for the knife, especially when the pain you feel is severe and relentless. However, these problems often have a muscular cause, and if this is the case, you may have the power to elimi-

nate that factor. Keep in mind, bones don't move themselves. Even when you have a technically correct diagnosis like scoliosis, bulging disks, or a compressed nerve, such spinal problems are often caused or greatly exacerbated by tightening of the muscles or fascia or by muscular weakness. This is where a good understanding of the paraspinal muscles, their actions, their attachments, and their influence on the spine can be helpful. Myofascial trigger points in these muscles can cause some of these common conditions or make them worse. For example, some of the deeper paraspinals attach to the side wings (transverse processes) of the vertebra. When they have trigger points, they can pull on the vertebra and tip them away from neutral.

For some people, the muscles on one side of the spine can become chronically tight. When this happens, the muscles on the other side sometimes give in, allowing

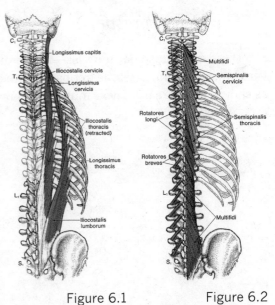

Figure 6.1   Figure 6.2

the spine to be pulled to the side with the tighter muscles. Many muscles, including some of the paraspinals, the iliopsoas, and the quadratus lumborum, attach to the vertebrae. And because the iliopsoas muscles attach to the disks between the vertebrae and the vertebrae themselves, the disks can also be pulled or pushed out of place by chronic muscular tension. We find that treating this is often very effective at restoring balance to the spine itself. By treating the muscles harboring trigger points and addressing any underlying perpetuating factors, it's possible to reduce the impact of conditions that misalign, tip, or rotate the vertebrae, spinal column, or pelvis (Travell and Simons 1999).

Where Are the Paraspinals and What Do They Do?

The paraspinals are a group of back muscles made up of a set of superficial longer muscles (the erector spinae) that run parallel to the spine, and a set of deeper, shorter muscles that run diagonal to the spine. The erector spinae include the longissimus thoracis, iliocostalis thoracis, and iliocostalis lumborum, as shown in figure 6.1. These longer muscles merge into a large, tendinous mass at the attachment to the pelvis at the sacrum. The shorter, deeper paraspinals include the multifidi, semispinalis, and rotatores, as shown in figure 6.2.

The Superficial Paraspinals

The superficial paraspinals (sometimes called the erector spinae group) consist of two parallel groups of muscles on each side of the spine running from the pelvis to the base of the skull. The closest to the spine is the longissimus group, and the group that is a bit farther out from the spine is called the iliocostalis group (see figure 6.1). Notice how these long muscle groups are composed of shorter muscle groups, many of which attach to the ribs. Trigger points in these muscles can affect the position and alignment of the spine. If one group is short, it can pull the spine to that side.

The Deep Paraspinals

The deep paraspinal muscles—the semispinalis, multifidi, and rotatores—run from vertebra to vertebra, and from vertebrae to ribs, or in the lumbar region, from vertebrae to the sacrum and pelvis, as shown in figure 6.2. These muscles run on a diagonal and can affect the position and alignment of each vertebra.

Functions of the Paraspinal Muscles

Acting together, the deep and superficial spinal muscles extend the spine. That means if you bend forward to pick something up, contraction of these muscles allows you to straighten up again or arch back. When one side acts by itself, they can also rotate the spine and torso, helping you bend sideways. The erector spinae help maintain upright posture and aid in making small adjustments as you move while standing or sitting. They also assist in breathing, as when coughing. Altogether, the paraspinals work to counteract gravity and the shortening of the abdominal muscles. As we age, we're in a constant battle against gravity pulling us forward and downward and often end up with hunched-over shoulders and a head-forward posture.

Paraspinal Pain Referral Patterns

Trigger points in the paraspinals can cause pain so intense you'd swear you were being stabbed. You might need to hold on to a table to stand up. The pain can be so intense that people become panicky. This sometimes causes heavier breathing and more severe pain and anxiety, and may eventually prompt you to go to the emergency room.

While the illustrations provided show the referred pain from trigger points at specific positions along the spine, note that trigger points can occur at any position along the spine. Here, we'll take a look at those with particular relevance for the low back. Figure 6.3 shows two possible trigger point locations in the longissimus thoracis that refer pain downward into the upper and lower buttocks. Trigger points in the middle part of the iliocostalis thoracis, shown in figure 6.4, can refer pain down to the upper buttocks, into the abdominals, and even upward into the shoulder. Trigger points in the iliocostalis lumborum,

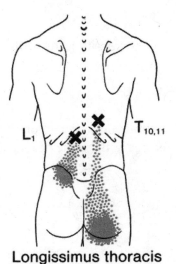

Longissimus thoracis

Figure 6.3

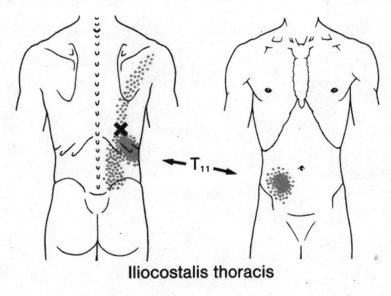

Iliocostalis thoracis

Figure 6.4

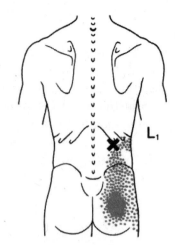

Iliocostalis lumborum

Figure 6.5

the lowest part of this muscle group, can refer pain into the low back and the mid to lower buttocks, as shown in figure 6.5. Closest to the spine and attaching between each vertebra, the multifidi and rotatores can cause spot-specific pain over and next to the spine anywhere from the head to the tailbone and into the buttocks, as shown in figure 6.6, which illustrates two specific examples, not all the possible locations.

Referred pain caused by any particular muscle in the deep paraspinals is usually located near the trigger point itself. Remember that trigger points can occur at any level of the deep paraspinals, from the neck down to the tailbone. For example, trigger points in one or more of the multifidi in the lumbar region can refer pain to the tip of the tailbone and make it supersensitive to pressure, and can also refer pain into the abdomen and down into the buttocks and upper thigh, as shown in figure 6.7.

When trigger points in the multifidi are activated, the pain can be so debilitating that it can put you flat on your back for days. Even slight rotational movements can be excruciatingly painful. Since referred pain from the deep paraspinals is very close to the spine and often severe, it can lead you (and your physician) to the conclusion that exploratory surgery or a surgical intervention is necessary. But if the pain is caused primarily by trigger points in the deep paraspinals in the first place, spinal surgery is unlikely to bring lasting relief. Wouldn't it be better to rule out muscular causes before resorting to surgery, with its risks and costs, in terms of both time and money? If trigger points are at the root of your problem, the self-care techniques in this chapter can help you reduce this pain so you can reclaim your health—and your life (Travell and Simons 1999).

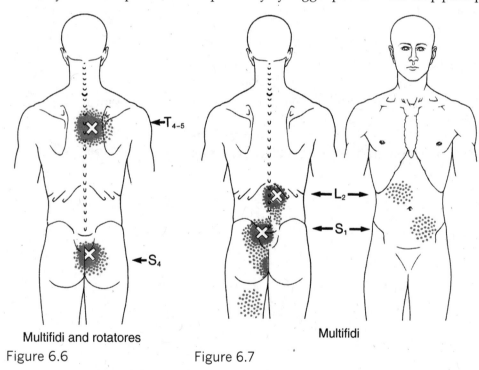

Multifidi and rotatores

Figure 6.6

Multifidi

Figure 6.7

What Aggravates the Paraspinals?

A number of things can cause problems in the paraspinals, including many common everyday activities:

- Sudden overload, such as when lifting, pushing, or pulling a heavy object, or when catching yourself from falling

- A fall from a height or a car accident with sudden impact

- Repetitive overuse of the paraspinals due to activities such as leaning over for a long time, bending down repeatedly, or not taking breaks when performing demanding tasks like painting or loading packages

- Quick awkward movements such as bending, twisting, or reaching, especially if the muscles have been overworked

- Any of the general perpetuating factors discussed in chapter 17

- Poor work ergonomics or poor seated posture, including while driving

- Tight hamstrings, which can pull the pelvis downward, shortening your stride and overloading the paraspinals

- Head-forward posture

- Chronically shortened abdominal muscles, which can pull the torso into a hunched-over posture, overloading the paraspinals

- Long periods of sitting or general immobility

- High stress in general

- Referred pain from the latissimus dorsi, serratus posterior inferior, rectus abdominis, quadratus lumborum, or iliopsoas, which can cause satellite activation in the paraspinals (the first two muscles listed aren't covered in this book)

Do I Have Trigger Points in My Paraspinals?

A number of symptoms point to trigger points in the paraspinals:

- Pain anywhere in the back or buttocks

- Difficulty or pain with any spinal movement, either arching the back or bending forward or to the side

- Difficulty or pain when getting up from a chair or low couch

- Restricted range of motion, with or without pain, in such activities as putting on or tying your shoes

- General weakness in the back

- Difficulty standing up straight or climbing stairs

- Steady and deep aching pain in the spine on one or both sides

- Trigger points in the gluteal muscles due to referred pain from the deep lumbar paraspinals

- Difficulty finding a comfortable position due to deep aching pain in the back

- Difficulty getting in or out of a car

- Sharp pains in your back so severe that you're forced to crawl on all fours

- Spot-specific pain near one of the vertebrae

Simple Tests

Two simple tests can help determine whether you have trigger points in your paraspinal muscles: the standing toe touch and the standing torso rotation.

Standing Toe Touch

This tests whether you have trigger points in your paraspinals, but it also tests for restriction in the gluteus maximus, hamstrings, and soleus, so it can't point conclusively to dysfunction in any of these muscles in particular. If you fail this test, you'll need to do more testing to pin down the source. Stand in your bare feet and, while keeping your abdominal muscles relaxed, slowly bend forward with your knees locked and see how close to your toes you can reach with your fingertips. If you experience pain, stop at that point and measure from there. If you're forty or younger and your hamstrings are in good condition, you should be able to touch the floor with the tips of your fingers. Give yourself an inch gap for every decade above forty. If you can't reach that far, even with our age allowance, or if you feel pain in your back, your buttocks, or the back of your thighs or lower leg when you do it, assume you have trigger points in one or more of the paraspinal muscles or in your gluteus maximus, hamstrings, or soleus.

Standing Torso Rotation

This movement tests the deep paraspinals. Stand about a foot away from a wall with your back facing the wall and your feet pointing straight ahead. Twist around to the right and try to touch both hands to the wall behind you, as shown in figure 6.8. Repeat this test to the left. If you can't do this, as shown in figure 6.9, or if you feel pain near your spine while doing it, you probably have trigger points in your deep paraspinals. Note that in figure 6.9, the torso isn't able to rotate, while in figure 6.8 the center of the chest is rotated much farther toward the wall.

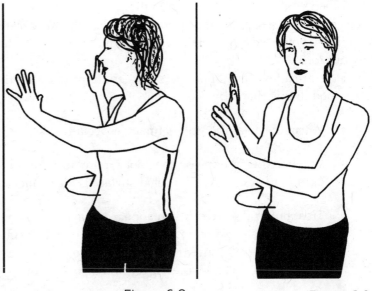

Figure 6.8   Figure 6.9

Helpful Hints for Eliminating Trigger Points in the Paraspinals

Together with self-care treatment to the areas marked in figure 6.10, there are some simple things you can do to alleviate or prevent trigger points in the paraspinals:

- Don't maintain any single position (seated or standing) for a long period, especially if your work is physically demanding. Do the range of motion exercises for the paraspinals in chapter 16, and incorporate some of them into your daily routine. This is one of the most important ways to help your paraspinal muscles.

- Use heat in the form of Mother Earth Pillows or Fomentek bags on your back and abdominal muscles, several times a day if necessary.

- When you are free of pain, perform gentle, progressive strengthening exercises for all of your torso muscles. A large fitness ball is good for this purpose.

- Make sure you're in an upright, neutral, supported, and relaxed position when seated.

Self-Care Treatment

In our experience, postural asymmetry caused by dysfunction in the quadratus lumborum, iliopsoas, and abdominals often needs to be addressed before treating the paraspinals. By treating these other muscles first, you can often eliminate postural asymmetry. Then when you get to the paraspinals, trigger point compression will be much more effective.

When you apply compression to the paraspinals, it's essential that you also treat the abdominals (see chapter 7), which are the opposer muscles for the paraspinals. To maintain a sustained pain-free condition, you need to maintain strength and flexibility in the muscles in both the front and the back of your torso.

Here are a few general pointers to keep in mind for all the compression techniques and stretches described in this chapter:

- Warm the area prior to treatment, especially when your symptoms are severe.

- When sitting or lying on the floor for any form of self-care (compression, stretching, range of motion exercises), a carpeted surface is ideal; alternatively, you can use an exercise mat.

- Treat both sides, even if you appear to have trigger points on only one side. The two sides are synergists and often work together to do the same job, so trigger points often develop on both sides. Or after trigger points develop on one side, the other side may overwork to compensate, causing new trigger points to develop.

- Refer to the MYO compression illustration (6.10) and compress all areas indicated by X's. The larger circled X's represent likely spots for trigger points, but the entire muscle requires treatment.

- Never exceed a pain level of 6 on a scale of 0 to 10.

- When applying compression, sustain the compression for up to 30 seconds and repeat at least two or three times, or until there's a noticeable decrease in pain and increase in range of motion.

- Gradually increase the amount of compression as you feel the muscle softening and relaxing. Be aware of how the tissues respond to treatment.

- When stretching, hold the position for two to three normal breaths.

- When a stretch is repeated several times on both sides, alternate sides with each repetition.

- After treatment and stretching, do the range of motion exercises for the paraspinals in chapter 16.

Compression

With the paraspinal muscles, it's especially important to match the level of compression to what you can comfortably tolerate. If you're in severe pain to begin with, start by applying heat with Mother Earth Pillows or Fomentek bags.

For guidance on self-compression, look at figure 6.10. The smaller X's represent all the areas where you should apply compression. The larger circled X's represent the most likely places to find trigger points. The T with a number next to it denotes the thoracic spinal level and the specific vertebra in that segment; L denotes lumbar spinal vertebrae; and S denotes vertebrae in the sacrum (which are fused in adults). Look for trigger points, taut bands, painful areas, and areas that won't stretch or contract in all the paraspinal muscles from top to bottom. Because there are so many paraspinal muscles and some of them overlap, figure 6.10 shows only half the areas to be treated; you need to treat the same areas on the opposite side, too.

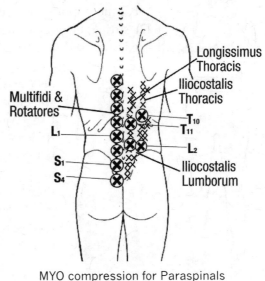

MYO compression for Paraspinals

Figure 6.10

Beginner Level: Standing Compression Against a Wall

Stand a short distance from a wall, facing away from the wall, and press your back into a softly inflated compression therapy ball. Remember to relax into the ball as you do this. If this doesn't provide enough compression, move your feet slightly away from the wall and lean more of your body weight into the ball, or further inflate the ball to make it firmer.

You can also use a tennis ball inside a knee-high stocking, as shown in figure 6.11. Hold the end of the stocking and drop the ball over your shoulder, then apply pressure by simply leaning against the ball on a wall, breathing slowly as you do so. Again, cover the entire area shown in figure 6.10. You may find it easiest to start near your spine just below the bottom of your shoulder blade and work your way down in parallel tracks. As you begin a new track, move outward away from the spine about an inch each time. Prolong the compression for two long breaths on any spots that are painful or tender.

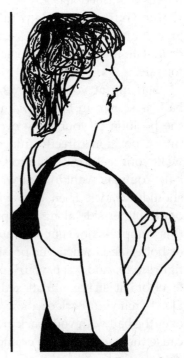

Figure 6.11

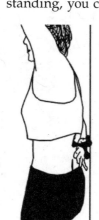

Intermediate Level: Treatment with the Backnobber or Jacknobber

For more spot-specific compression, use a Backnobber while standing (as in figure 6.12), sitting, or lying down. This tool also offers the advantage of being easily positioned and used in different ways. If you're in too much pain to treat yourself while standing, you can sit down or use it to treat your back while lying in bed. You can also use it with a warm Fomentek bag by pressing through the warm bag. Another adaptation would be to rest on a warm pack like a Mother Earth Pillow first, then apply compression using the Backnobber. Another option for intermediate-level compression is to use a Jacknobber against a wall. Place the tool between your back and the wall right next to your spine and just below the bottom of the shoulder blade and work your way downward. At each location, gently press your back against it as shown in figure 6.13. Hold this for one breath, then use your hand to reposition the tool to another place along the muscle.

Figure 6.12   Figure 6.13

Advanced Level: On the Floor Using a Compression Therapy Ball

Once you're comfortable with the treatment techniques described above, you're ready to apply compression to your paraspinals with a ball while on the floor. Start with a 7-inch compression therapy ball and inflate or deflate it as necessary to achieve a firmness you can tolerate.

Starting at your buttocks, slowly roll up onto the ball, as shown in figure 6.14, using your feet to control the position of your body over the ball. Work the ball into a position directly under your lower spine, then walk your feet forward to roll your body down over the ball. You may want to stop when you get between your shoulder blades. Then start again, with the ball out to either side along the spine. While doing this compression, support your head with one or both hands whenever possible, as shown in figure 6.15, and keep your spine straight and level, or if it isn't painful, flexed slightly forward. Don't arch your back or allow your body to rest over the ball with your back arched, as this may cause the paraspinals to cramp. For a variation

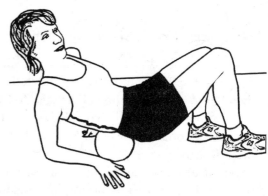

Figure 6.14

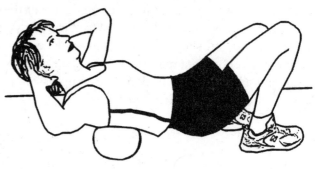

Figure 6.15

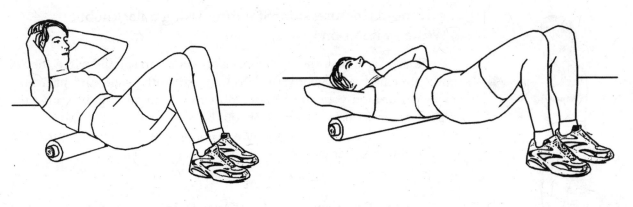

Figure 6.16   Figure 6.17

that you may find easier and more stable, try using a 4-inch foam roller while lying on your back, as shown in figures 6.16 and 6.17.

If this technique causes more than moderate pain (6 on a scale of 0 to 10), go back to a more gentle form of compression. Or if it's too hard on your abdominal muscles, turn over and treat them as described in chapter 7. After using more gentle methods, give the advanced techniques another try to see if you can tolerate them.

Advanced Level: On the Floor Using a Backnobber

For more spot-specific compression, use a Backnobber while lying on your back on the floor, as shown in figure 6.18. Use the floor as your fulcrum and press upward with the least force needed to achieve good compression. If the pressure is too strong at first, you can use a rubber band to hold a washcloth over the knob of the tool until you're able to tolerate the pressure. For an even more advanced compression, cross your right leg over the left and let both legs and your hips fall toward the left, as shown in figure 6.19. This will stretch the paraspinals on your right side. Slide the Backnobber under your back and press into the muscles along the spine on your right side. After treating the entire right side, shift your legs to the other side and treat the paraspinals on the left side.

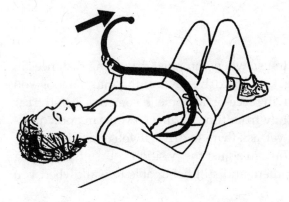

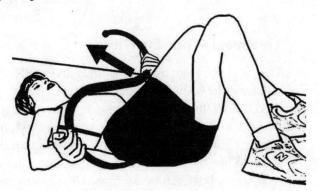

Figure 6.18   Figure 6.19

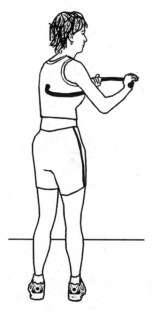

Advanced Compression: Standing Using a Backnobber While in Rotation

Another way to use the Backnobber on your paraspinals while they're slightly stretched is to gently twist your torso to the right and bring the Backnobber around your torso under your right arm, placing it against the paraspinal muscles on the left side of your back. Use your right hand to press outward (toward the right) on the end of the tool, as shown in figure 6.20. Experiment with different degrees of stretch and rotation.

Figure 6.20

Advanced Compression: Bent Over Using a Backnobber

We strongly recommend using the Backnobber while bent over at the waist in a seated position. (You can also do this while standing, but seated is less stressful.) This is another position that puts the paraspinals in a stretched position while you apply compression, which is the most effective way to apply compression. This position also gives you a great deal of control.

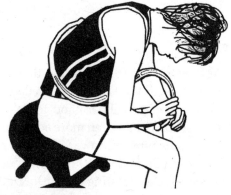

While seated, bend over at the waist and support the weight of your torso by resting your elbows on your thighs, as shown in figure 6.21. Remain relaxed in your abdomen and hips. Bring the Backnobber around your waist and press into the end of the tool in front of you with both hands. With the end that's pressing into your back, follow a line just next to the spine, looking for taut bands and painful spots, then work your way outward at about 1-inch intervals. Experiment with different positions, such as tipping your pelvis forward or backward or gently arching your spine or leaving it straight.

Figure 6.21

Treatment While Driving

The Jacknobber (or a tennis ball) is an excellent tool to use when you must drive long distances in pain. Place it between your back and the driver's seat back as you drive. By leaning into the tool, you can accomplish the same compression you would while lying face-up at home. If someone is in the car with you, ask them to adjust the position of the tool slightly from time to time so you can apply pressure to the entire area of the tightened muscles, or better yet, ask them to drive. If you're driving alone, it's better to use the tool while parked at a rest stop, so you can adjust the position yourself. On a long trip, the Jacknobber can be an invaluable aid to getting there and still being able to walk when you arrive.

Stretching

For the superficial paraspinals, anything you can do to bend your torso forward can serve as a good stretch, and anything to come up from that bent-over position will act as a contraction. Remember to keep your abdominal muscles relaxed while you bend over. If you're not sure they're relaxed, press a hand into your abdomen as you bend over to feel whether the muscles are contracting. The cat back and old horse exercise (see the exercises for the paraspinals in chapter 16) is particularly helpful for the paraspinals. You can enhance these stretches by shifting your hips from one side to the other.

The deep paraspinals stretch and contract as the torso is twisted and bent. You can stretch these muscles by simply twisting around in your chair from one side to the other and back. When you twist to the right, you contract the muscles on the right side and stretch the muscles on the left, and vice versa. Here are instructions for beginner stretches for the paraspinals.

Seated toe touch

While seated in a chair, bend forward, reach down to your feet, and touch the floor, as shown in figure 6.22. Keep your abdominal muscles relaxed. To contract the paraspinals, sit up tall and breathe deeply. Then repeat the stretch, this time reaching back through your legs a bit if you can.

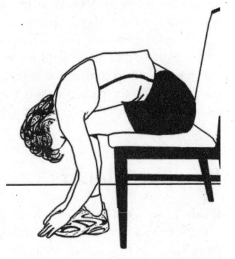

Figure 6.22

Single leg to chest

While lying on your back, bring one leg up toward your armpit on the same side and squeeze your knee to your chest, as shown in figure 6.23. Keep your abdominal muscles completely relaxed and grasp your leg behind your thigh, not over your knee.

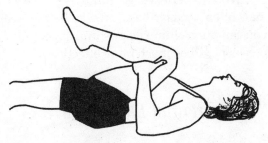

Figure 6.23

Double leg to chest

From the same starting position, grasp the backs of both thighs and use your arm strength to pull both legs up to your chest, raising your buttocks and tailbone off the floor if you can. Again, keep your abdominal muscles relaxed.

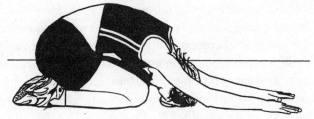

Figure 6.24

The child's pose

This stretch gets its name from a popular yoga pose. Sit on your heels, lean forward with your torso on your thighs and your forehead resting on the floor, and stretch your arms out in front of you, as shown in figure 6.24. If your knees hurt or you can't rest your buttocks on your heels, you can put a pillow between your heels and your buttocks. If you can't get into this position due to lack of flexibility in the thighs, this may indicate trigger points in your quadriceps muscles, in the front of the thigh.

Contracting and Relaxing

Many techniques can help contract the paraspinals. Seated rotation contracts the rotatores and multifidi. First rotate as far as you can without pain in one direction and hold the position for two breaths, then relax and repeat on the other side. To add variation, lean back slightly while you do this rotation.

Two exercises described in the paraspinals protocol in chapter 16 also contract the paraspinals: the cat back and old horse series and the seated pelvic tilt series. If you have a friend to work with, try the exercise for seated contraction of the abs in chapter 7 (page 105). Another good way to contract and then further stretch the paraspinals is the standing toe touch. Each time you bend to touch your toes, the paraspinals stretch, then contract to bring you back up again.

For Practitioners

While it may seem best to simply start treating the back muscles to eliminate patients' low back pain, it's important to do a complete evaluation first to determine which muscles are the primary cause of their pain. Taking a full history will help you uncover any perpetuating or precipitating factors. When you hear their symptoms and complaints, you'll form a clearer idea of the likely reasons for their pain.

In our experience, postural asymmetry caused by the quadratus lumborum, iliopsoas, and abdominals often needs to be addressed before treating the paraspinals. By treating these other muscles first, you can often eliminate postural asymmetry. Then when you get to the paraspinals, trigger point compression will be much more effective.

Differential Diagnoses

This book is concerned with the myofascial component of low back and buttocks pain. As stated in the introduction, we encourage people with low back pain to consult their primary care physician to rule out nonmyofascial causes of pain. However, it's not uncommon for chronic back pain to result from a combination of causes, none of which alone justify surgical intervention. In these circumstances, the myofascial component is often completely overlooked, and if other approaches aren't effective, the patient is left to suffer unending pain. In these cases, it's helpful for you to know about such factors as lumbar facet syndrome or sacroiliac syndrome, which can be a major component in back pain. It's also critically important that you understand the many myofascial and nonmyofascial elements that may interact with each other. Particularly with referred pain from the paraspinals, there's a greater possibility of this combined causation than with other types of low back pain. Your ability to work proactively with other practitioners may make a real difference for your patients.

Treatment Techniques

When patients are in acute pain, it may be almost impossible for them to tolerate much stretching or manual compression of any kind. In these circumstances, your first task is to desensitize the painful areas. Warm Fomentek water bags or Mother Earth pillows may be helpful, and spray and stretch treatment can be particularly useful. It's also imperative to limit the amount of time you have the person in any one position. Vary positions and use support bolsters and pillows for their comfort. Use heat, especially when stretching and immediately after spray and stretch treatment.

Stretching, Contracting, and Relaxing

We like to have the patient alternately stretch, contract, and relax the muscles being treated at almost any time during treatment. Contraction allows us to more easily find taut bands of fibers and determine the ability of certain muscles to contract and relax upon demand. For the paraspinals, contraction and relaxation can be done in any of the treatment positions we outline below. Unless patients are in unbearable pain, they should be able to raise one or both arms or legs or their entire torso at least slightly from a prone position. If they can do any of these, have them hold the position for just a few seconds, then relax. Feel for the stabilizing function of the paraspinals and note any rigid or denser areas. Also feel for hypotonic or flaccid areas and feel for the coordinated exhalation-relaxation phase. Does it take a long time for the muscles to relax after the brief contraction? Is there twitching or cramping? These are obvious signs of dysfunction and good reason to continue treatment.

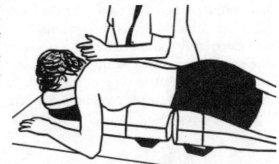

Figure 6.25

Treatment Positions

To begin treatment, we usually start with warm Fomentek bags under the patient lying prone on a body support system. We palpate the superficial paraspinals, then we may use a forearm to compress larger areas of these muscles, as shown in figure 6.25, looking for and treating any taut bands and trigger points we find. We then may use the tip of the elbow, as shown in figure 6.26, to apply compression to the deeper paraspinals. Since so many other muscles can influence the spinal muscles and posture, during a complete session we turn the patient onto their side and treat the quadratus lumborum, abdominals, and iliopsoas on as much of a stretch as the patient can comfortably tolerate (see chapters 8, 7, and 5). Then we place the patient in a supine

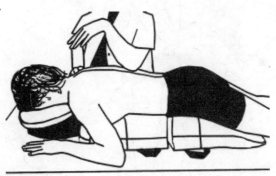

Figure 6.26

position and once again treat the abs and iliopsoas in as much of a stretched position as can be comfortably tolerated, with warm Fomentek bags beneath the shortened paraspinals. Be careful not to leave the patient too long in this position, as the paraspinals can become activated. Continually monitor the patient's perception of tightness in their back. Have the patient turn onto one side and crunch up their knees to their chest to stretch the back before getting up.

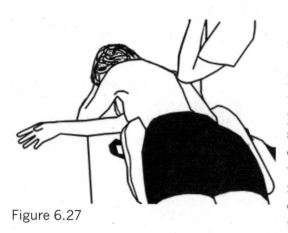

Figure 6.27

Here are a few other positions that are effective for treating the paraspinals.

Prone position with a rotational component: Separate the body support cushions and have the prone patient place their right arm under and across their chest, as shown in figure 6.27. If you don't have body support cushions, place pillows beneath the patient's neck and waist. These positions allow you to treat all the torso muscles on the stretch. Treat the multifidi and rotatores on the right side, looking for taut bands of tissue and treating any that you find. Then reverse the position and treat the muscles on the opposite side.

Prone position with a lateral torso curve: In this position, the patient's torso and legs are curved to the left to present the paraspinals on the right side in a stretched position, as shown in figure 6.28. Maintain this position only as long as the patient is comfortable. Reverse the position and treat the opposite side. Placing the patient in a stretched position generally makes it easier to identify taut bands.

Standing stretched and bent over the treatment table: In this position, it's important to make sure the degree of torso flexion is comfortable for the patient. An adjustable treatment table (preferably with electrically controlled height adjustment) is ideal for this purpose. Or you can use a folded body support cushion with a warm Fomentek water bag, as shown in figures 6.29 and 6.30, or pillows, as shown in figure 6.31, to support the upper body. In figure 6.31, the patient is comfortably relaxed over the treatment table while compression is being applied through a warm Fomentek bag. An alternative is to apply compression through a heated Mother Earth Body Wrap, as shown in figure 6.32.

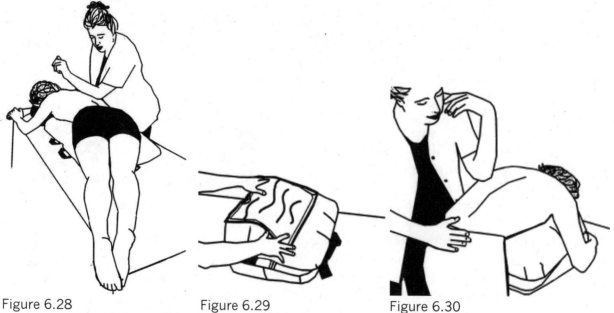

Figure 6.28   Figure 6.29   Figure 6.30

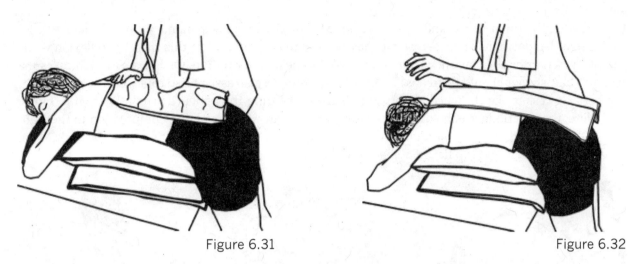

Figure 6.31   Figure 6.32

Standing stretched and bent over the treatment table with a rotational component: Have the patient bring one arm across and under their chest, with their shoulder and the side of their face on the table, as shown in figure 6.33. With the left arm under the chest as shown, treat the left (stretched) side of the back. Then reverse the position and treat the opposite side.

Sitting on the treatment table flexed: Have the patient sit on the table with their torso flexed and legs straight in front, as shown in figure 6.34. This position allows almost ideal access to the paraspinals in the stretched position for a variety of treatment techniques, including manual compression, spray and stretch (described below), and stretching, contracting, and relaxing.

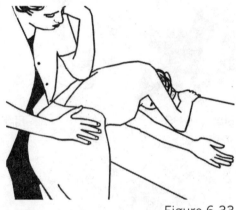

Figure 6.33

Sitting on the treatment table flexed with rotation: Have the patient sit on the treatment table with their torso flexed and rotated, as shown in figure 6.35. This position isn't a good choice in early stages of treatment, as the patient may be in too much pain to permit such flexion and rotation of the torso. However, when the patient can comfortably assume this position, it allows superb access to the deep paraspinals in the stretched position and is ideal for any of the treatment techniques noted above.

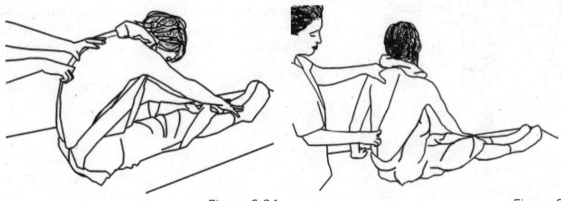

Figure 6.34   Figure 6.35

Sitting with the torso flexed and/or rotated on a stool or chair: For patients with tight hamstrings, the straight-leg positions described above may be very uncomfortable. In this case, torso flexion while seated in a chair or stool, as shown in figure 6.36, can be a better option. Of course, in such cases the patient's hamstrings should be treated in due course. You can also assist torso rotation (thereby providing better access to the stretched deep paraspinals) by holding the patient's arm, as shown in figure 6.37. Here, the practitioner is holding the patient's right arm while applying compression to the right side of the spine with the patient rotated to the left. Figure 6.38 shows this position from the back. Make sure the abdominals and hip flexors remain relaxed.

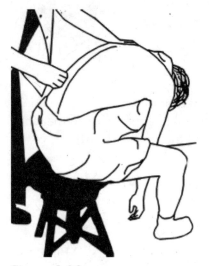

Figure 6.36

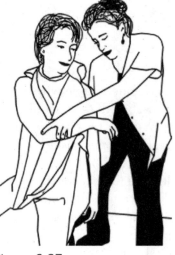

Figure 6.37

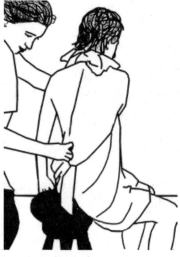

Figure 6.38

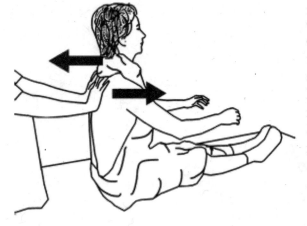

Figure 6.39

Active seated torso extension: In this position (on either the table or the floor), the patient attempts to extend their back against resistance provided by the therapist, as shown in figure 6.39. After at least 10 seconds, the patient exhales and relaxes the effort, keeping their abdominal muscles relaxed, then reaches forward as the therapist provides a gentle assist from behind, as shown in figure 6.40. Bear in mind that tight hamstrings or gluteal muscles, which are very common, can restrict the degree of stretch and may need to be addressed later in treatment.

Advanced Treatment Techniques

The following treatment techniques and positions can be used at a later stage of treatment, when most of the patient's pain has dissipated and normal muscle flexibility has been restored. After completing treatment of the paraspinals and abdominal muscles to ensure there's no major myofascial dysfunction or pain, you can treat the paraspinals in a shortened position. Have the patient assume a modified cobra pose using either their elbows or pillows for passive torso extension, as shown in figure 6.40. Begin compression at the lowest lumbar segment and work your way up from there.

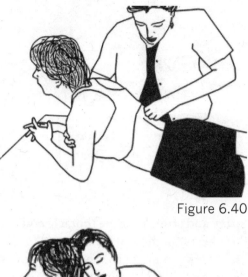

Figure 6.40

The cobra pose can be modified by having the patient extend their arms to elevate the torso, keeping the back muscles and abdominals as relaxed as possible. Place one hand on the rectus abdominis on either side and just below the belly button, and press inward with gentle pressure, as shown in figure 6.41. You're looking for painful taut bands that won't stretch. At the same time, use the thumb or first and second fingers of your other hand to press into the erector spinae of the low back at approximately the same level. Work your way down to the pubic bone and sacrum and allow the patient to rest as needed. Then begin compression at the belly button again and work your way upward to the sternum and mid back. This is a highly effective way to treat two key opposer muscles in their respective stretched and shortened positions. Don't try this advanced technique until the person has almost

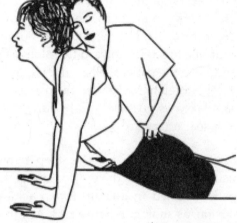

Figure 6.41

normal range of motion in the paraspinals, otherwise the muscles may lock up when placed in this shortened position.

Spray and Stretch

Spray and stretch can be remarkably effective for the paraspinals because it gives you the opportunity to cover a large area in a relatively short time. Review the general guidelines for spray and stretch techniques in chapter 2. And remember that for patients whose abs and iliopsoas are chronically tight, it's generally a good idea to treat those muscles before treating the paraspinals. After all of the spray and stretch treatments outlined below, have the patient move through the full range of motion at least three times (see the standing twist and bend series in the paraspinals protocol in chapter 16).

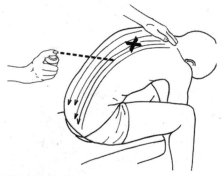

Figure 6.42

Seated spray and stretch: Have the patient sit in a chair and bend over, with their arms between their legs, as shown in figure 6.42. Start between the shoulder blades and spray downward to the upper buttocks. Run the sweeps along both sides of the spine. Next, apply heat to the area you just sprayed and allow the patient to completely relax; then ask them to bend farther into a stretched position, and repeat the spray technique. Depending on the patient, it may be necessary to also treat the abdominals and iliopsoas (on the table; see chapters 7 and 5), as those muscles can become activated while in this shortened position.

Spray and stretch for the thoracic and lumbar erectors: Have the patient sit on the treatment table with their legs straight. Have them bend forward, drop their head, hunch their back, and reach toward their toes. Begin spraying as the patient slowly exhales, starting at the mid-scapular region and extending downward as far as the buttocks. Be sure to spray along both sides of the spine. Instruct the patient to continue to stretch toward their toes as you spray the vapocoolant. Apply heat immediately afterward and have the patient relax fully while you gently push their upper torso forward to achieve a slightly greater stretch. Make sure the patient keeps the abdominal region as relaxed as possible, and be sure to address the abdominals and iliopsoas afterward.

Spray and stretch for the deep paraspinals: This technique is usually done after the erector spinae have been treated. With the patient seated in a chair, try to achieve both torso rotation and flexion, as shown in figure 6.43. Ask the patient to turn toward the side with the pain. Spray the muscles starting at the thoracic spinous processes and continue with short sweeps angled downward and outward. Apply heat immediately afterward, and encourage the patient to fully relax and allow the stretch to go a bit farther.

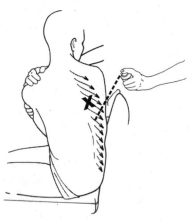

Figure 6.43

Summary

As you may notice, we offer a greater variety of positions and treatment options for this muscle group than for any other in the book. This is because there are so many different muscles in the paraspinals, and because the nature of those muscles lends itself to treatment in so many different ways.

Because of the severity of pain associated with chronic tightening of the paraspinals, encourage your patients to learn and use the self-care protocols described in this chapter, and keep some self-treatment tools on hand so you can instruct patients in their use. Daily treatment is usually needed to gain the upper hand with pain due to trigger points in the paraspinals, so your patients will benefit greatly from self-care.

Chapter 7

Rectus Abdominis

The abdominals comprise many muscles that when dysfunctional can aggravate or cause low back pain. Trigger points in them refer pain to various parts of the body. But only the rectus abdominis—which we'll refer to simply as the abs—refers pain directly to the back, so it will be our primary focus.

Fortunately, it's easy to rule the rectus abdominis in or out as a cause of pain, and it's one of the easiest muscles to treat. The rectus abdominis is often the focus of intense effort in the quest for "six-pack" abs; however, this devotion to vanity can result in chronic contraction of the abs, and back pain as a result. That said, deconditioned abdominal muscles can be problematic too. As is often the case, moderation is the key.

Where Are the Abs and What Do They Do?

The abs attach at their upper ends to the outer surfaces of the fifth, sixth, and seventh ribs (and more rarely, the fourth or even third rib) and go straight down to the top of the pubic bone, as shown in figure 7.1. They contain three or four tendinous ridges called *inscriptions*, and the right and left sides are divided by a vertical line of connective tissue called the *linea alba*. This vertical line and the three (or sometimes four) horizontal inscriptions form the "six-pack" configuration of the muscle in a well-conditioned (or overconditioned) person.

The abs help bend the torso forward and are obviously used during sit-ups or abdominal crunches. They help maintain stability when we stand erect, and they work harder when we're climbing than when walking on flat ground. When the back muscles are also contracted, the abs assist in a number of more basic functions, including coughing and defecation, as well as childbirth.

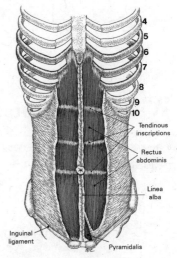

Figure 7.1

Rectus Abdominis Pain Referral Patterns

The abs can develop trigger points within each divided segment, but only trigger points below the lowest tendinous inscriptions refer pain to the low back. This region is right above the pubic bone (see the lower trigger point in figure 7.2) Trigger points here refer pain across the low back, the upper buttocks, and the sacroiliac joint (where the sacrum joins the pelvis), and can also cause spasms of the urinary sphincter. Trigger points on one side of the abs can refer pain across the entire low back.

Another important region is just to the side and slightly below the belly button in the lower abdomen, as shown in figure 7.3. Trigger points here can cause pains similar to appendicitis, premenstrual symptoms, and severe menstrual cramping and pain, and also cramping and pain throughout the abdomen that's made worse by movement. These trigger points can even cause diarrhea and, more rarely, pain in the genitalia.

The third area likely to contain trigger points is along the inside edge of the rib cage near the upper attachments of the abs (the upper trigger point shown in figure 7.2). Trigger points here cause pain running horizontally across the mid back and sometimes a feeling of heartburn. Referred pain from these trigger points often causes satellite trigger points in the paraspinal muscles (Travell and Simons 1999).

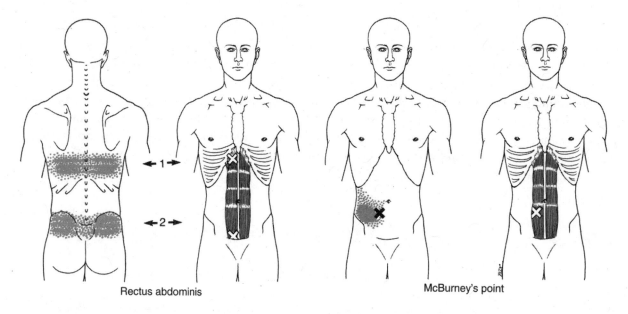

Rectus abdominis

McBurney's point

Figure 7.2   Figure 7.3

What Aggravates the Abs?

The most common cause of trigger points in the abs is too much sitting, especially in a slumped-over, head-forward posture. Other perpetuating factors include the following:

- Doing too many sit-ups or overexercising in general

- High stress and emotional tension

- Straining during bowel movements or during prolonged labor

- Scar tissue caused by surgery

- Improper bending while lifting a heavy object (bending over from the waist rather than from the knees and not relaxing the abs while bending)

- Too much abdominal fat, restricting torso movement

- Chronic tightening of the abs to suck in your gut and look thinner

- Wearing tight belts, control-top panty hose, or tight girdles

Do I Have Trigger Points in My Abs?

The presence of low back pain *across* the back is one indicator of trigger points in the lower abs. Other telltale signs are abdominal weakness, reduced range of motion, painful menstrual cramps, heartburn, and abdominal pain and cramping in general. Another indicator is increased pain in your lower back upon taking a deep breath. Here are a few simple tests for trigger points in the abs.

Palpation Test

Start by looking at figure 7.4. The larger X's show the most likely spots for trigger points that may cause back pain. To do this test, lie flat on your back. Starting just above the pubic bone, press into the rectus abdominis with your fingers or knuckles, as shown in figure 7.5, then release. Taut bands will feel firmer than adjacent tissue. Move gradually upward and repeat the compression until you're at the top of the muscle, as shown in figure 7.6. Do this on both sides and note any areas that are firmer than the surrounding tissue or tender, or that cause pain in the back or elsewhere when you press on them.

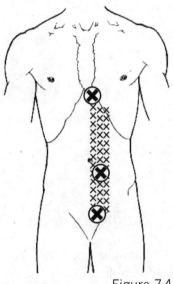

Figure 7.4

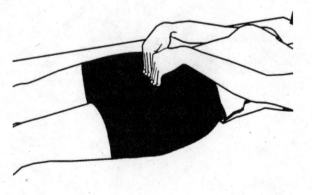

Figure 7.5

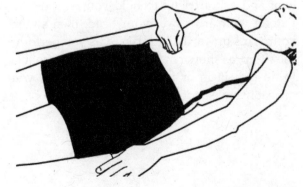

Figure 7.6

Contract and Feel Test

The contract and feel test looks for muscle weakness or an increase or decrease in pain upon compression. Ask a friend to gently press into your abs as you lie on your back. Note any areas that are painful, and ask your friend to identify any that are denser or harder than surrounding muscles. (If you have considerable abdominal fat, this may be difficult for an untrained person to do.) Next, while your friend releases the pressure, raise your legs about 6 inches off the floor to contract your ab muscles, then have your friend gently press into any sensitive abdominal areas. If your pain increases during this compression, this tends to confirm the presence of trigger points in the abs. If your pain decreases with this compression, the pain may originate in organs in the abdominal cavity, so you should consult a physician.

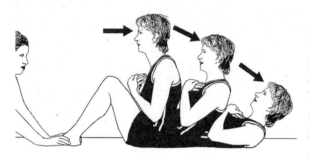

Figure 7.7

Abdominal Roll-Down

The abdominal roll-down tests the strength of the abs. Assume a seated position on the floor with your knees bent and ask a friend to hold your feet down. With as little strain as possible, roll your torso backward and down to the floor gradually over 10 seconds, as shown in figure 7.7. If you can roll down slowly without pain, your rectus abdominis is probably fine. If you can't roll down slowly because it's too painful or your abs begin to quiver as you lower your torso, you probably have trigger points in your abs.

Swing Arm Sit-Up

Another good strength test for the abs is to do an abdominal sit-up using your arms for momentum. Lie on your back with your knees bent and ask a friend to hold your feet down. Extend your arms over your head, then swing your arms upward and forward as you perform the sit-up, as shown in figure 7.8. If you're unable to do the sit-up or feel pain as you do it, you probably have abdominal trigger points.

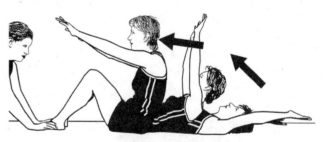

Figure 7.8

Postural Tests

Trigger points can cause chronically shortened or weak muscles that impair your ability to stand in a comfortable, pain-free, erect posture. While in your natural standing posture, ask a friend to check you for any of the following conditions, which can indicate chronically contracted abs or weak paraspinals or abs:

- Forward-leaning or head-forward posture

- Arms or hands rolled inward

- Loss of the normal curve in your lower back (a flat low back area)

- An excessive lumbar curve or a large, protruding belly

- The front of the ribs pulled down and mid back area rounded

- Shoulders and chest moving up and down while breathing

Next examine your seated posture and consider the following questions. Answering yes to any of them indicates chronically tight abs:

- Do you tire quickly when you sit upright?

- Do you tend to lean forward and rest your elbows on your knees or desk?

- Do you maintain a head-forward posture?

- Do you feel more comfortable slouching forward?

- Do you lean back and sit on your upper buttocks rather than your lower pelvis?

Finally, examine your posture while walking or ask a friend to watch you as you walk. If any of the following apply to you, you probably have chronically tight abs, and possibly other chronically tight muscles, as well:

- A bent-forward posture

- A head-forward posture

- Taking smaller than normal steps

- Keeping your pelvis frozen in one position as you walk

Helpful Hints for Eliminating Trigger Points in the Abs

In addition to self-care treatments, there are a few simple things you can do to help alleviate trigger points in your abs:

- If you sit for long periods, take frequent breaks to stand, walk, and stretch. Consider using a standing desk.

- Consciously relax your abs throughout the day. Keep your neck and chest relaxed while breathing, and allow your abdominal muscles to expand as you inhale. In general, try to breathe more slowly.

- Avoid sleeping in the fetal position, flat on your back, or on your stomach. If you sleep on your back, place a pillow under your knees. Lying on your side is best, but don't allow your knees to creep up toward your chest. (See chapter 17 for more on sleep positions.)

- Let your belt out a few notches, and don't wear control top panty-hose or a tight girdle.

Self-Care Treatment

The key region of the abs that refers pain into the low back is the lowest part, just above the pubic bone. But an important caveat is needed: In many people, the entire abdominal group is chronically contracted, with trigger points throughout the muscle, because so many of us sit for most of our waking hours. You can't get rid of trigger points in the lowest part of the muscle without relieving contraction in the rest of the muscle as well, so it's best to do compression, stretching, contraction, and range of motion exercises for the entire rectus abdominis. And whenever you treat your abs, it's also important to stretch your back muscles. In fact, if the abs need treatment, you should also read chapter 6, Paraspinals, and follow the recommendations there.

We prefer to treat the abs on the stretch, meaning you're draped over pillows while lying face-up to elongate the ab muscles as you treat them. **Caution:** If you've been diagnosed with bulging or herniated lumbar disks, check with your doctor before stretching your abs in this way.

The stretched position shortens your back muscles, so if you're in this position for any length of time, it's important to stretch your back afterward. A good way to do so is to turn over onto your side, then grasp your knees to your chest as in figure 7.9. Then roll over to an all-fours position and get up. For the same reason, anytime you treat your abs on the stretch, afterward do a few repetitions of the cat

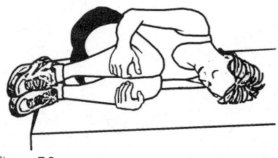

Figure 7.9

back and old horse exercise (see the exercises for the rectus abdominis in chapter 16). The child's pose, shown in figure 7.10, is another good way to lengthen the back muscles while relaxing the abs.

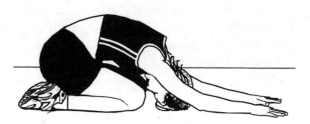

Figure 7.10

Here are a few general pointers to keep in mind for all the compression techniques and stretches described in this chapter:

- Warm the area prior to treatment, especially when your symptoms are severe.

- When sitting or lying on the floor for any form of self-care (compression, stretching, range of motion exercises), a carpeted surface is ideal; alternatively, you can use an exercise mat.

- Treat both sides, even if you only appear to have trigger points on one side. The two sides are synergists and often work together to do the same job, so trigger points often develop on both sides. Or after trigger points develop on one side, the other side may have to overwork to compensate, causing new trigger points to develop.

- Refer to the MYO compression illustration (7.4) and compress all areas indicated by X's. The circled X's represent likely spots for trigger points, but the entire muscle requires treatment.

- Never exceed a pain level of 6 on a scale of 0 to 10.

- When applying compression, sustain the compression for up to 30 seconds or longer and repeat at least two or three times, or until there's a noticeable decrease in pain and increase in range of motion.

- Gradually increase the amount of compression as you feel the muscle softening and relaxing. Be aware of how the tissues respond to treatment.

- When stretching, hold the position for two to three normal breaths.

- When a stretch is repeated several times on both sides, alternate sides with each repetition.

- After treatment and stretching, do the range of motion exercises for the rectus abdominis in chapter 16.

Compression

For guidance on self-compression, look at figure 7.4. The smaller X's represent all the areas where you should apply compression. The circled X's represent the most likely places to find trigger points. However, since you need to normalize the entire length of the muscle, we recommend that you treat the entire muscle, from top to bottom, applying more sustained compression to any areas that are firmer or more painful. If you have especially tender or tight abs, apply heat first, using a warm Fomentek bag or a long Mother Earth Body wrap, as shown in figure 7.11. A warm bath or a dip in a hot tub is also a great idea. You can also try using a superficial distraction technique. This can be as simple as using a sugar or salt scrub, soft brush, or loofah while slightly stretching your abs in the tub or shower. You could also try using an Orbit Massager on your abs, either while standing or while lying on your back, as shown in figure 7.12.

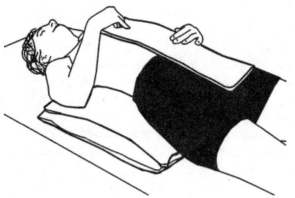

Figure 7.11

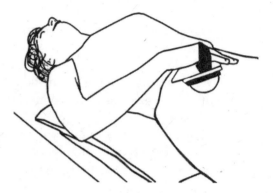

Figure 7.12

Stretched Positions to Enhance the Effectiveness of Compression

Depending on the extent of tightness in your abs, it may be difficult to stretch them very much at first, even though that's the best position for compression. However, you can stretch your abs to some degree simply by compressing them while you lie on your back in a neutral position.

Here's a progression of increasingly stretched treatment positions. Start at whatever level you can without undue pain and discomfort, and don't progress through these positions too quickly or proceed to the next position before you're able to do so without pain. After a few days or weeks in each position, you should be able to move on to the next. From the various stretched positions described below, select the greatest stretch you can achieve with only mild discomfort, and hold that position for no longer than 3 minutes while treating your abs as described below:

1. Lie flat on your back with your arms at your sides, then lift your arms over your head. Notice how this adds to the stretched feeling in your abdomen. You can keep one arm overhead and use the other to apply compression.

2. Lie on your back with one pillow under your low back.

3. Lie on your back with one pillow under your low back and with one arm over your head.

4. Add another pillow beneath your back to further arch your back and stretch your abs.

5. Add a third pillow.

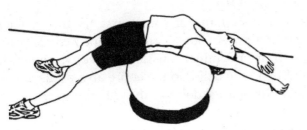

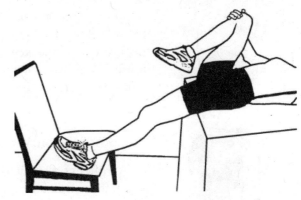

Figure 7.13

6. Lie draped over a 65-centimeter fitness ball with a base for stability, as in figure 7.13. You may want to have a friend support you until you gain confidence. You can also anchor your feet at the baseboard of a wall while doing this stretch.

Figure 7.14

7. Lie on a bed or treatment table with one leg hanging over the end, supported by a chair, as in figure 7.14.

8. Next, try letting both legs hang over the end, supported by a chair, as in figure 7.15.

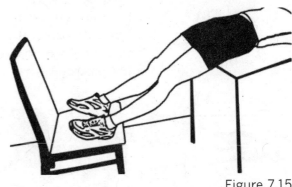

9. Finally, try the same position, but with a lower chair or step stool to support your legs.

Figure 7.15

Be sure to get up and out of these positions by rolling onto your side, then bringing your knees to your chest. Then do some cat back and old horse stretches (see the exercises for the abdominals in chapter 16) to stretch your back muscles and relax and shorten your abs.

Compression While Lying Face-Up

Of all the muscles covered in this book, the abs are perhaps the easiest to treat with your own hands. Starting just above your pubic bone, press into your abs with your fingers, as shown in figure 7.5, above, or with your knuckles, or with self-care tools such as a Jacknobber, a Knobble, or an Orbit Massager. Use one hand to help the other hand press in. Apply compression on both sides, moving gradually up the muscle looking for painful spots and taut bands of muscle. When you locate one, press in and hold for at least 10 seconds. An alternative is to grab the skin above a painful area and pinch it for 10 seconds, then roll the tissue between your fingers and thumb. This method ensures that the superficial layer of abdominal fascia is healthy and pliable. If it's initially too painful to apply compression to your abs, try massaging the whole abdominal region gently using long gliding strokes with a lotion or cream.

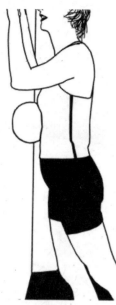

Figure 7.16

Compression While Standing

If the positions above are too stressful for you at first, try this position instead: Stand facing a wall and press your abs into a 7-inch compression therapy ball while keeping your abdominal muscles relaxed, as shown in figure 7.16. Move slowly and press the ball into the entire area of the abs on both sides, from the bottom of the rib cage down to the pubic bone.

Compression While Lying on Your Side

Another good way to apply compression to the abs is while lying on your side with your head supported by your lower arm or a pillow. Bring a 7-inch compression therapy ball toward your belly and roll partially onto it, as shown in figure 7.17. Slowly put as much of your weight as you can tolerate onto the ball, while at the same time trying to relax and melt into the ball. Look for painful, taut bands of muscle, and when you find them, hold the compression for at least 10 seconds. Then continue to move the ball until you've treated the entire muscle on that side. Treat both sides, and repeat the compression, holding it for a longer period (as much as 25 seconds) in areas that feel more sensitive or painful. Notice any referred pain in your back as you do this compression. Don't worry; this is simply a confirmation that you have trigger points in your abs.

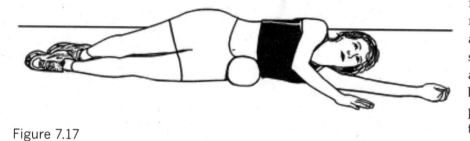

Figure 7.17

Advanced Compression on the Floor

If you're following the entire self-care protocol, over a couple of weeks you should become less sensitive to compression of your abdominal muscles and the overlying fascia. This is the time to advance to the next level.

Start face-down over a 7-inch compression therapy ball at your pubic bone on one side of your abs, resting your body weight on the elbow on that side while you bend the knee of the opposite leg, as shown in figure 7.18. This allows you to stretch your abdominals while controlling the amount of weight you place over the ball. Slowly glide your body downward so that the ball moves along your abdomen all the way up to your rib cage. Relax and feel the muscle and fascia lengthening. If this is too challenging at first, you

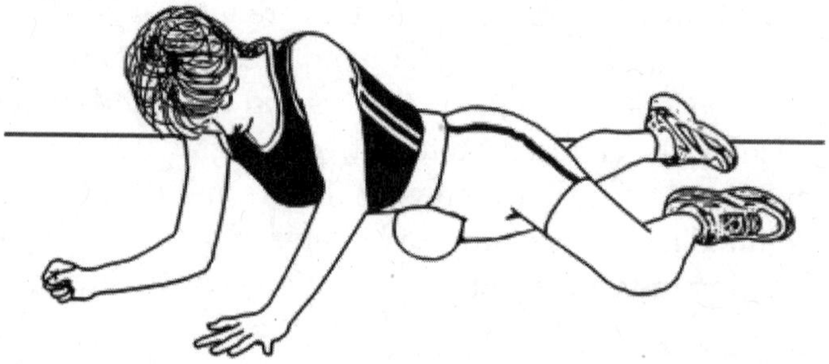

Figure 7.18

can use pillows or a rolled-up blanket, as shown in figure 7.19, to support part of your body weight so you don't place as much weight on the ball at first.

For a more advanced technique, place the ball at your pubic bone as you hold your torso up using your arms while keeping both legs straight, as in figure 7.20. Slowly glide your body downward by extending your arms, as shown in figure 7.21, so the ball moves along your abdomen all the way up to your ribs. Remain relaxed and try not to contract your abs as you apply compression.

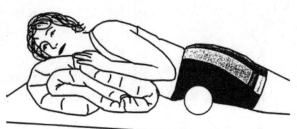

Figure 7.19

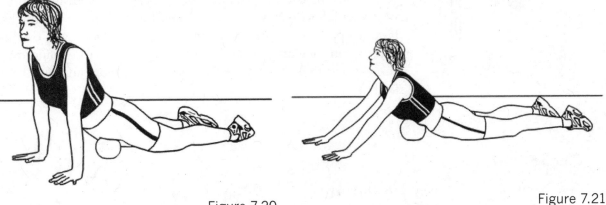

Figure 7.20

Figure 7.21

Stretching

Almost all the treatments described above contain some element of stretching. Here are some different abdominal stretches that can be done as a variation or in addition to those described above.

Lunge with Backward Bend

While standing, step forward with one leg and lean back onto the other leg, as shown in figure 7.22. (You can hold on to a countertop or sturdy chair for stability.) Hold the stretch for 10 seconds, and do it at least twice on each side. This also stretches the iliopsoas. Vary this technique by leaning straight back at first, then leaning to one side and then the other.

To add contraction and relaxation while you're in this position, have a friend press against the front of your shoulders as you contract your abs by attempting to bring your rib cage downward. Hold this resistance for 10 seconds, then relax as you exhale and lean farther back while still lunging. Repeat on the other side.

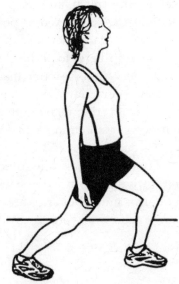

Figure 7.22

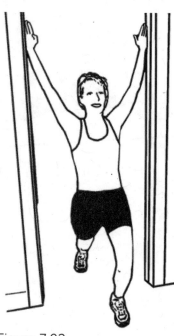

Figure 7.23

Standing Body Stretch

Place your forearms on the doorjambs on either side of a doorway as high as you can. This elevates your rib cage and lengthens the front of your torso. Step forward with one leg, and as you put your weight on the front leg, bend your torso backward as far as you comfortably can, as in figure 7.23, and hold for 10 seconds. Repeat this at least twice, then repeat the stretch with the other leg forward. If your chest muscles are tight, you may not be able to stretch your abs fully in this position. In this case, just stretch as far as you can without discomfort. As you stretch, note which areas are most sensitive or painful. These areas need further treatment. This stretch benefits all the muscles in the front of your torso, from your shoulders down to the pubic bone and even into your thighs. If your upper chest muscles (your pectorals) are too tight, do this stretch with one arm on the doorjamb at a time. To enhance this stretch over time, bend your front knee a bit more and lean back farther.

Cobra Stretch

Don't attempt the advanced stretch shown in figure 7.24 until your back pain is almost gone and you've been able to do the other stretches in this chapter with virtually no pain. Start with a passive version of the stretch, simply lying face-down on one, then two, then three pillows placed under your chest. Allow your body weight to deepen the stretch, and keep your abs and low back muscles as relaxed as possible. We've seen advanced yoga students with severe back pain who were still able to perform this stretch. Upon close observation, we found that they were unconsciously contracting the back muscles. This prevented them from relaxing those muscles in the shortened position, and actually caused trigger points and chronic tightening of the deeper muscles of the low back.

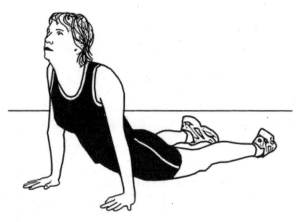

Figure 7.24

After you've passively stretched your abs with pillows in the cobra position, do the exercise actively. Start by lying flat, face-down with your hands beneath your shoulders. Gradually raise your torso with your arms until your arms are completely straight, as shown in figure 7.24. Hold for at least 10 seconds, then gradually let your torso down, keeping your back and abdominal muscles completely relaxed.

Contracting and Relaxing

These exercises use movement against resistance alternating with relaxation to help you achieve greater mobility. Alternating these exercises with the stretches described above will lead to more improvement in mobility than stretching alone. It's most effective to do these exercises with a partner. Once you've eliminated trigger points in your abs, you can resume a regular fitness routine, including "cheater" sit-ups with an arm swing (see figure 7.8, above), traditional sit-ups, or even crunches on a 65-centimeter fitness ball.

Seated Contraction of the Abs

As you sit on a chair, have your partner hold the front of your shoulders while standing behind the chair. Try to bring your rib cage down against your partner's resistance by contracting your abs, as shown in figure 7.25. Hold this contraction for at least 10 seconds, then exhale and relax. Next, to contract the paraspinal muscles (the opposers to the abs), have your partner restrain your upper back with their hands as you push your whole upper torso backward against the resistance. Hold this for at least 10 seconds, then exhale and relax. Perform the entire sequence three times.

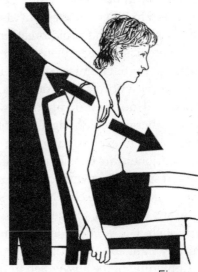

Figure 7.25

Abdominal Roll-Down Contraction

This exercise starts in the traditional sit-up posture on the floor. With your knees bent and a partner holding your feet, roll slowly backward (see figure 7.7, above) until your torso is on the floor. This both strengthens and lengthens the abs. When you finish, lie back, relax, and stretch your arms over your head for at least 10 seconds. To get back to the starting position, roll to one side and push yourself up with your hands. Perform this exercise five times, and increase reps over time.

Contracting the Opposer Muscles

It's essential that you treat the opposer muscles, in this case the erector spinae (see chapter 6, Paraspinals), when you treat the abs. The only way to maintain a sustained pain-free condition in the torso is to maintain strength and flexibility in the muscles in both the front and back of the torso. To this end, you may want to alternate the abdominal roll-downs with the superman exercise (see the exercises for the paraspinals in chapter 16).

For Practitioners

A careful distinction must be made in discussing problems in the rectus abdominis: Trigger points in this muscle can cause a host of problems that have nothing to do with low back pain. We want to acquaint you (and your patients) with these problems, because patients may have them and mistakenly assume there is some other, nonmuscular cause.

Differential Diagnoses

A surprising number of symptoms may be caused by trigger points in the rectus abdominis, and this can lead you down the wrong path. Trigger points in the rectus abdominis can produce not only referred pain in other muscles, but also other disorders, accounting for such conditions as paradoxical breathing, shallow and rapid breathing, anxiety, heartburn, diarrhea, severe menstrual pain, constipation, anorexia, nausea, retention of urine, groin pain, and colic in babies. These trigger points can also cause pain that mimics pain due to angina, appendicitis, gynecological diseases, peptic ulcer, and irritable bowel syndrome. We don't mean that trigger points in the abs always cause these conditions—but when they do, they are almost always overlooked. Therapists and physicians need to consider the possibility that muscular trigger points may be at the root of many worrisome symptoms that might otherwise lead to expensive, risky, or unnecessary medical testing and treatment. So when clients or their practitioners are considering antacids, laxatives, or stronger prescription drugs for these various abdominal symptoms, why not first test for and treat any myofascial component of the condition? If the symptoms go away, the client will be spared the need for drugs or other medical procedures.

In terms of causes, trigger points in the rectus abdominis can develop as a result of postsurgical trauma, such as C-section delivery and scarring. Prolonged emotional stress also can contribute to chronically tight abs. Practitioners need to consider how disease or emotional or physical trauma may cause tightening of the abs, which in the long term can lead to the development of trigger points, myofascial dysfunction, and serious physical symptoms, as noted above. These simple connections are very often lost in the labyrinth of modern medical testing and diagnosis.

If the abs contain trigger points and taut bands of tissue, it can be hard for the person to lift their rib cage. Chronically shortened abs lead to a slumped-over posture, rounded shoulders, and poor breathing habits. In this posture, people tend to breathe shallowly, only into the upper chest and neck, instead of expanding the diaphragm and breathing into the abdomen. Shallow, rapid breathing often leads to chronic hyperventilation, overbreathing, and trigger points in other muscles involved in breathing.

Treatment Techniques

Side-Lying with Body Support

Because supine treatment can be too much for the patient at the beginning, it's best to start treatment with the patient lying on their side on a body support system. (Refer back to figure 2.1 to see the setup for this with warm Fomentek bags.) This positioning supports the patient's head, neck, and chest; provides space for the shoulder, and gives support under the waist that allows the rectus abdominis, obliques, and quadratus lumborum to stretch.

Treating the Rectus Abdominis and the Paraspinals Together

Although we generally recommend treating muscles in as much of a stretch as the patient can comfortably tolerate, treating the rectus abdominis on the stretch puts the erector spinae in a shortened position. To prepare them to be in this position, we often treat the paraspinals on the stretch first, then treat the abdominals on the stretch, then treat the paraspinals on the stretch again. Having the patient stand bent over the treatment table, as described in chapter 6, Paraspinals, is an excellent position for quickly treating the back muscles.

Lying on the Treatment Table with Legs on a Chair

After treating the paraspinals, treat the abs on the stretch. If you don't have the rectus abdominis stretched while applying compression, you may actually go through and into the muscles and viscera beneath them. In addition, in the stretched position the taut bands and trigger points will stick out because they won't stretch, making it easier to find the problem areas.

Have the patient sit at the foot of the treatment table. Arrange the body support cushions and pillows where the patient's waist and head will be. Put a warm Fomentek bag on top of the pillows where the low back will lie. Now cradle the patient's torso, and gently lower them down onto the warm Fomentek bag. Place their feet on a chair. To add more stretch, move the chair away till the legs are straight (see figure 7.15, above). If this stretch is too painful, place a warm Fomentek bag on top of the abs, sandwiching the patient in warm water. Treat the abs through the warm Fomentek bag with your elbow, as shown in figure 7.26, starting an inch above the pubis and working slowly up to the rib cage. We often use the tip of the elbow to compress trigger points against the pubic bone and the pubic symphysis. We usually try to add to the stretch during treatment by putting the patient's arms over their head. Always treat bilaterally, even if the pain and tightness are mainly on one side. To add more stretch, take the foot of the side you're treating off the chair and let it stretch farther down.

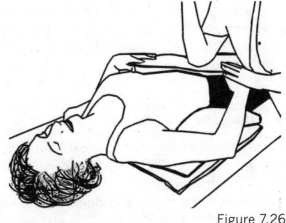

Figure 7.26

Next, use oil or cream and apply gliding strokes over the entire abdomen. If the patient winces with even light pressure, try using vapocoolant spray, as described below.

Ending this stretch properly is important. First, bring the patient's arms down to their sides and ask them to relax. Lightly massage the abs as you reduce the degree of stretch. Now put their feet on the chair with their knees bent. Continue massaging the abs while asking the patient to breathe and relax. Then place one hand on the abs and one hand behind the upper back and assist the patient in rising to a seated position. Have them flex forward to contract their abs. If they can, have them bring their chest to their thighs and rest there for a moment as you apply light gliding strokes to lengthen the longissimus thoracis and iliocostalis lumborum, which will have been shortened throughout treatment.

Next, assist the patient in standing, then have them lean over the table, with pillows under the abs and chest. This will allow you to treat the back again.

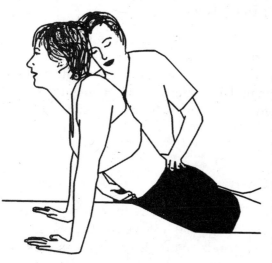

Figure 7.27

Advanced Treatment Position: Lying Face-Down

Start with the patient lying prone over a body support system to slightly stretch the paraspinals, with warm Fomentek bags under the abs to warm them before treatment. First spend a few minutes treating the paraspinals, then ask the patient to come up on their hands and knees briefly so you can remove the body support cushions. Have the patient lie down prone again, then come up on their elbows as they lift their torso gradually while keeping their hips on the treatment table. Reach under the torso and look for taut bands in the rectus abdominis. As the abs relax and lengthen, increase the stretch by having the patient come up onto their hands, as shown in figure 7.27. This really brings out the taut bands because the stretch is so extreme. Use your fingers to look for painful taut bands from origin to insertion of the rectus abdominis, and treat by pressing up into the painful taut bands. If the patient tires of this position, give them a mini break. Be sure to treat bilaterally, and when you're done, have the patient perform several repetitions of the cat back and old horse exercise (see the exercises for the abdominals in chapter 16), or have them turn onto their side and bring their knees to their chest to stretch the back muscles and contract the abs.

Spray and Stretch

Spray and stretch can be very helpful in restoring full range of motion to chronically tightened abdominal muscles. With the patient lying supine in a stretched position, with one leg outstretched and the other supported, as shown in figure 7.28, start spraying at the sternum. Spray downward toward the pubic bone in slow parallel sweeps as indicated by the lines in figure 7.28. As you complete each sweep, remind the patient to stay relaxed and to exhale as the spray starts. The vapocoolant will feel cold, so to avoid involuntary tensing make sure the room temperature is warm. After you've completed the spray and stretch, apply heat over the area to help further relax the abs in the stretched position. Afterward, always bring the patient's knees to their chest for a few moments. Repeat the entire procedure with the other leg stretched off the table and the previously stretched leg now bent and supported. Afterward, have the patient move through their full range of motion at least three times using some of the exercises in the abdominals protocol in chapter 16.

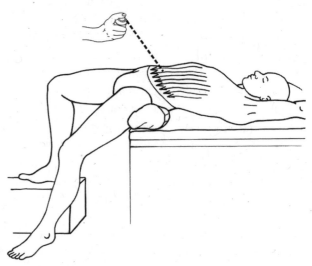

Figure 7.28

Chapter 8

Quadratus Lumborum

Travell and Simons called the quadratus lumborum the joker of low back pain. However, there's nothing funny about low back pain, and the good doctors didn't intend a joke. They may have meant that this muscle isn't easy to find and treat and that, covered as it is by other muscles, it's often overlooked. They also may have been referring to how the severity of pain caused by chronic contraction of this muscle sometimes leads physicians to diagnose nerve root compression as the probable cause and recommend surgery as the most appropriate remedy. In fact, the quadratus lumborum alone is often the sole cause of low back and buttocks pain. Based on our clinical experience, we put it near the top of the list of all muscles referring pain to these areas.

An important aspect of this muscle is that, contrary to common practice, it's most effectively treated while you're lying on your side and in a stretched position. It's more difficult to treat from the back or front because it's buried under other muscles. Chronic pain caused by the quadratus lumborum can be so disabling that you may need to be treated by a therapist at first. Unfortunately, few therapists treat it in the side-lying position, so take this book along to help your practitioner understand how to treat this muscle most effectively.

Where Is the Quadratus Lumborum and What Does It Do?

The quadratus lumborum forms part of the back wall of the abdomen. It attaches to the lowest (twelfth) rib, the transverse processes of the upper lumbar vertebrae, and a portion of the iliac crest, as shown in figure 8.1.

This muscle plays a role in respiration, assisting in coughing and forceful exhalation. When one side works alone, it enables you to lean over to that same side or lift the

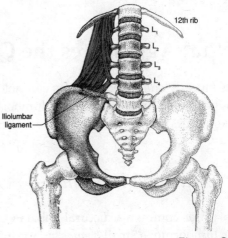

Figure 8.1

hip on that side. When you're seated or standing and the quadratus lumborum muscles on both sides contract together, they allow you to arch your back. This muscle also helps stabilize the lumbar spine when you're standing or seated.

Quadratus Lumborum Pain Referral Patterns

The quadratus lumborum has two trigger point regions (see figures 8.2 and 8.3). The white X's show the most likely places to find trigger points; dots show the pain referral patterns. Trigger points in the superficial (outer) layer cause pain in the upper and lower hip, buttocks, and in the abdomen, near the appendix. Trigger points in the second area, deeper in the torso and closer to the spine, cause pain over the lower buttocks and mid-buttocks over the sacroiliac joint, where the sacrum joins the pelvis.

When this muscle is severely contracted, it not only causes excruciating pain, it can also stick out to the side like a knife edge when you're lying on your side. In such cases it's impossible to lie on that side. Referred pain from the quadratus lumborum can also cause activation of the paraspinals, the iliopsoas, the abdominal obliques, and the latissimus dorsi muscles (the last two of which aren't covered in this book). Referred pain from the quadratus lumborum can also cause activation in the gluteus medius and gluteus minimus, leading to various secondary symptoms that mimic or may be mistaken for sciatica or disk syndrome (Travell and Simons 1992).

Quadratus lumborum trigger points and referred pain patterns

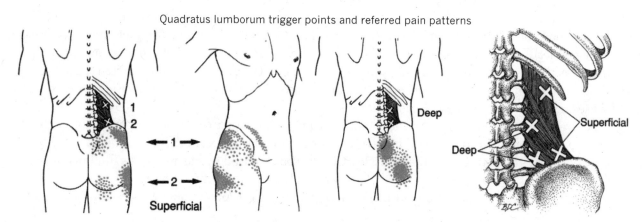

Figure 8.2

Figure 8.3

What Aggravates the Quadratus Lumborum?

Chronically shortened muscles can hold the pelvis in a fixed tilt to the back or the front, activating trigger points in the quadratus lumborum. In addition, structural imbalances in the body and bad ergonomics (at work or at home) can also aggravate this muscle.

Structural Imbalances

Three common structural imbalances, usually undetected, can cause trigger points in the quadratus lumborum: a small *hemipelvis*, meaning one side of the pelvis is smaller than the other; leg length inequality, meaning one leg is shorter than the other; and short upper arms in relation to the length of the torso, which can cause you to lean to one side to allow your forearm to reach an armrest. Fortunately, all these structural imbalances are easily corrected. For details, see Mechanical Factors, in chapter 17.

Bad Ergonomics

Anything that causes you to habitually lean to one side or the other can aggravate the quadratus lumborum; for example, an ill-fitting chair, lack of armrests, or armrests at the wrong height. This applies to car seats as well as chairs. An ill-fitting chair can also cause you to habitually slouch forward. Typing while looking to one side to see source materials is another culprit. Sleep positions can also be problematic. For example, if you always sleep on your right side, the right quadratus lumborum is lengthened and the left quadratus lumborum is shortened. (See chapter 17 for details on sleep positions.)

Do I Have Trigger Points in My Quadratus Lumborum?

Several common problems point to trigger points in the quadratus lumborum muscles:

- You can't turn over in bed due to pain.

- You can't bear the pain of standing upright or walking.

- You have difficulty bending forward or leaning to either side.

- Coughing or sneezing is extremely painful.

- There is evidence of nerve compression due to vertebrae pulled sideways by a chronically contracted quadratus lumborum muscle.

- Chronically contracted quadratus lumborum muscles can lead to postural imbalances that ultimately result in migraine headaches, temporomandibular joint disorder, or other regional myofascial pain syndromes.

- Postural asymmetry may be due to trigger points in the quadratus lumborum.

- You experience deep aching pain even when immobile. This can be so excruciating while standing that you have to hold on to something for support.

- Slight movements of the lower back may cause sharp, stabbing pain.

- Severe trigger point activation can feel like a cramp or spasm and have you crawling on all fours.

- More rarely, you might also experience pain in the groin, scrotum, or testes, or pains down the hip and side of the thigh and into the ankle.

Nerve Compression

The quadratus lumborum attaches to the transverse processes of the lumbar vertebrae in the lower back. If these muscles are shorter on one side, they can actually pull on the sides of the vertebrae, which can tip the vertebrae on their sides and squeeze them closer together. In extreme cases, this can actually compress the nerve root. So a chronically shortened quadratus lumborum can cause true nerve root sciatica, because the root of the sciatic nerve exits the spinal cord through these openings. This sideways tipping of vertebrae due to taut bands in the quadratus lumborum can also compress the disk between the vertebrae and cause it to bulge outward.

Because of the severity of the pain this causes, surgery is sometimes recommended to take pressure off this intervertebral space. This is unfortunate, as myofascial trigger point treatment can alleviate these conditions. We've seen X-rays that prove it. Naturally, your physician must be your principal guide when you have a diagnosis of nerve compression or bulging disks. But you should consider the possible myofascial origin of the condition before consenting to surgery. From the standpoint of both cost and potential side effects, it makes sense to first eliminate myofascial causes before having surgery.

Drs. Travell and Simons said, "A finding of osteoarthritic spurs and/or some narrowing of the space between the lumbar disc spaces does not, by itself, establish the source of low back pain, since many people with moderate degenerative joint disease have no pain" (Travell and Simons 1992, p. 39).

Standing Side Bend Test

If you have one or more of the problems discussed above, here's an easy test to determine whether trigger points are present in the quadratus lumborum. When doing this test, look for reduced range of motion, weakness, or pain.

Stand up straight with your feet shoulder width apart and your palms flat against the sides of your thighs. Bend your torso to each side in turn, reaching your fingers down along your thigh toward the outside of the knee. Bend straight to the side; don't lean forward. Return to a neutral standing position, try the additional movements described below and answer the related questions:

- Are you unable to reach down to either side so the tip of your middle finger is at or below the top of your knee?

- Does it hurt in your low back and hips when you bend to either side or when you arch your back?

- Do you get relief from pain in your low back and buttocks if you put your hands on your hips and press down while standing or walking, as shown in figure 8.4?

- Is it painful or difficult to swing your hips from side to side?

- Do you have difficulty or pain in your low back and/or buttocks when you tilt your pelvis or hike up one hip?

If you answer yes to most of these questions, you probably have trigger points in your quadratus lumborum.

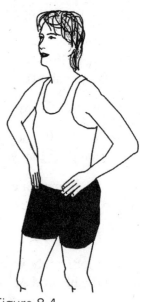

Figure 8.4

Helpful Hints for Eliminating Trigger Points in the Quadratus Lumborum

Beyond self-care treatments, there are several simple things you can do to help alleviate the pain of chronically contracted quadratus lumborum muscles:

- Sleep on both your right and left sides. Experiment with tilting your hips forward or backward as you lie on your side in bed. See which position is most comfortable, and use pillows to help you maintain that position while you sleep.

- Temporarily eliminate stress on your low back muscles when you're standing by putting your hands on your hip bones and pressing down on your hips and into your waist, as shown in figure 8.4, above.

- Use a low back support cushion while sitting or driving.

- Use a forward-tilting seat wedge when sitting for extended periods of time. This will help you tilt your pelvis forward.

- If you have short upper arms, use a chair with adjustable armrests to prevent you from leaning to one side or the other.

- Correct for leg length inequality by using a heel lift under the shorter leg. (See chapter 17 for details.)

- Correct for a small hemipelvis by sitting on a butt lift on the short side. (See chapter 17 for details.)

- Evaluate for and correct Morton's foot syndrome. (See chapter 17 for details.)

- Spend less time sitting, and take a break at least once every hour whenever you must sit for an extended time. During these breaks, do the exercises for the quadratus lumborum in chapter 16.

- Do as much of your work standing as possible.

- Correct uneven sitting surfaces of chairs, couches, or car seats.

- If you sleep on your back, place a pillow under your knees to prevent excessive shortening of the quadratus lumborum.

- If you sleep on your side, place a king-size pillow between your knees and lower legs, all the way down to your feet. It can also be very helpful to place a small pillow or even a warm Fomentek bag under your waist to keep the quadratus lumborum muscles in a neutral position.

Self-Care Treatment

Here are a few general pointers to keep in mind for all the compression techniques and stretches described in this chapter:

- Warm the area prior to treatment, especially when your symptoms are severe.

- When sitting or lying on the floor for any form of self-care (compression, stretching, range of motion exercises), a carpeted surface is ideal; alternatively, you can use an exercise mat.

- Treat both sides, even if you appear to have trigger points on only one side. The two sides are synergists and frequently work together to do the same job, so trigger points often develop on both sides. Or after trigger points develop on one side, the other side may overwork to compensate, causing new trigger points to develop. This is particularly important in treating the quadratus lumborum muscles.

- Refer to the MYO compression illustration (figure 8.5) and compress all areas indicated by X's. The larger circled X's represent likely spots for trigger points, but the entire muscle requires treatment.

- Never exceed a pain level of 6 on a scale of 0 to 10.

- When applying compression, sustain the compression for up to 30 seconds and repeat at least two or three times, or until there's a noticeable decrease in pain and increase in range of motion.

- Gradually increase the amount of compression as you feel the muscle softening and relaxing. Be aware of how the tissues respond to treatment.

- When stretching, hold the position for two to three normal breaths.

- When a stretch is repeated several times on both sides, alternate sides with each repetition.

- After treatment and stretching, do the range of motion exercises for the quadratus lumborum in chapter 16.

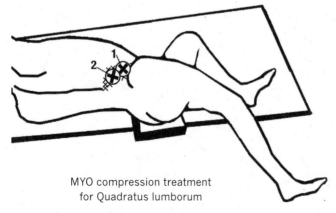

MYO compression treatment
for Quadratus lumborum

Figure 8.5

Compression

For guidance on self-compression, look at figure 8.5. The smaller X's represent all the areas where you should apply compression. The larger circled X's represent the most likely places to find trigger points. When treating the quadratus lumborum, you must press through the abdominal muscles. Compression can be achieved using your hands, a small inflated ball, a Backnobber, or a Jacknobber. While it takes strength to press into your own side, using the right self-care tools will make it much easier. It's best to treat this muscle in both neutral and stretched positions.

Start Gently

If your abs or quadratus lumborum are particularly tight or painful, try starting with an Orbit Massager. You can also use a nongreasy cream to massage your waist, or even light brushing. Focus on breathing slowly and relaxing the tight muscles. Using light massage and heat can help you relax sufficiently to permit some compression treatment. You can also refer back to chapter 3 for a refresher on

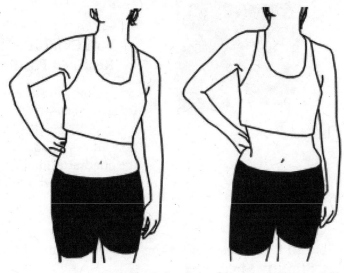

how to desensitize very tender or painful areas. If you're initially in too much discomfort to apply compression yourself, ask a friend to do it using their hands or elbows. Make sure they apply only as much pressure as you request.

You can use your own hands to pinch the skin above the quadratus lumborum, as shown in figure 8.6. Or you can press directly into your waist with your fingers or thumb, as shown in figure 8.7. But this technique can be difficult to sustain for long periods due to the strength required. So using self-care tools to provide compression to the quadratus lumborum is much preferred.

Figure 8.6   Figure 8.7

Ball Compression on the Wall

Try starting with a compression therapy ball placed between your waist and a wall. If the pressure is too much to begin with, deflate the ball a bit or use a larger ball. First, lean into the ball so it presses into your waist above the pelvis. Stretch the muscle slightly by raising the arm closest to the wall and slightly bending to the side opposite the ball, as shown in figure 8.8. Apply gentle compression and keep rolling slowly over the ball as you press into it, looking for tender and painful spots. When you find one, sustain the pressure for at least 10 seconds, and then gradually release it. This is a very effective way to begin compression treatment, as your reactions will tell you when you've found the right spots. Treat both sides, even if you suspect trigger points on only one side.

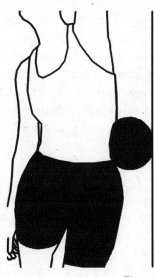

Figure 8.8

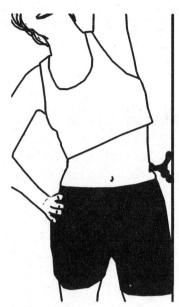

Figure 8.9

Using a Jacknobber Against a Wall

The Jacknobber is an excellent tool for treating the quadratus lumborum. The small surface area of the knobs allows you to apply more spot-specific pressure than with a ball. While standing next to a wall, place the Jacknobber on the wall just above your hip, as shown in figure 8.9, and gently press your waist into it, carefully controlling the amount of pressure into your side as you look for taut bands and painful spots. Next, stretch your body slightly away from the wall as you raise the arm closest to the wall over your head.

Ball Compression While Stretched in a Partially Reclined Position

Lie on your side with your weight supported by your elbow or forearm, thus stretching your waist. Now roll your waist slowly over a compression therapy ball, looking for painful spots. This position allows good control of how much compression you apply to the quadratus lumborum, and treating in a stretched position is less likely to cause shortening of the muscle.

Ball Compression on the Floor with the Quadratus Lumborum Slightly Shortened

Next, lie on your side and place a compression therapy ball against your side at your waist. With your arms above your head and resting on the floor, roll partially onto the ball, as shown in figure 8.10, again searching for tender or painful spots. Wherever you find them, relax into them using your body weight on the ball and hold for at least two relaxed breaths. Continue to roll the ball to different spots on the side of your abdomen above your pelvis and below your rib cage.

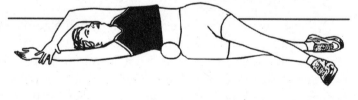

Figure 8.10

Using the Backnobber While Lying on Your Back

The Backnobber is also excellent for treating the quadratus lumborum. It allows you to apply more pressure than the Jacknobber, and in a very controlled way. As with the Jacknobber, the small surface area of the knobs allows you to apply pressure to very specific spots. Lie on your back and place the larger end of the Backnobber under your back a couple of inches out from the spine, as shown in figure 8.11. Position the tool under your back so it conforms to the curve of your waist and place the knob wherever you feel the greatest tightness and tenderness. In this position, it should apply almost no pressure. Next, press the free end of the Backnobber away from your body, starting very gently at first. Apply pressure gradually up to a level you can tolerate, hold the pressure for 10 seconds, and then gradually release it. When you find a spot that's particularly tender or painful, you can extend the compression to as much as 30 seconds, as long as you don't exceed a pain level of 6 out of 10. Move the tool up, down, and

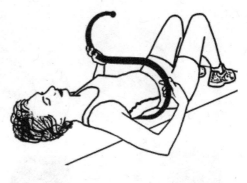

Figure 8.11

to either side, each time applying pressure about an inch or so from the previous position. You'll be able to tolerate more pressure in some spots than others. Use as much pressure on each spot as needed to reach the same level of tolerable discomfort. Even if you have pain on only one side, treat both sides.

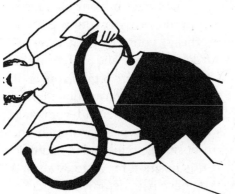

Figure 8.12

Using the Backnobber in a Stretched Side-Lying Position

Lie sideways over a pile of pillows, as shown in figure 8.12, to stretch the upper part of the quadratus lumborum. Use the Backnobber to press into the stretched side of your waist. Alternate leaning slightly forward and slightly backward as you apply pressure.

Stretching

Remember, stretching is more effective when combined with contraction and relaxation, so definitely include those elements, as described below, when stretching your quadratus lumborum.

Standing Stretch

This is the same as the standing side bend test for determining whether trigger points are present in the quadratus lumborum. Stand with your feet shoulder width apart and your palms flat against the side of your thighs. Bend your torso to each side in turn, reaching your fingers down along the side of your leg. Stretch as far as you can without discomfort. Hold the stretch for at least 10 seconds, then gradually return to an upright position. Repeat this stretch three times on each side, stretching just a little farther each time.

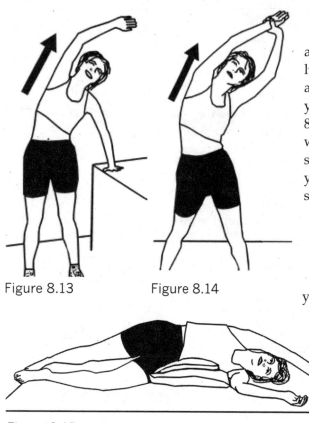

Figure 8.13   Figure 8.14

Advanced Standing Stretch

This stretch is good for other muscles in the abdomen and torso, in addition to the quadratus lumborum. Stand with your legs about 2 feet apart and lean gradually to the left side while reaching your right arm over your head, as shown in figure 8.13. If necessary, hold on to a sturdy table or chair with your left hand for support. To intensify the stretch, pull your right arm up and to the right with your left hand, as shown in figure 8.14. Repeat this stretch three times on each side.

Side-Lying Passive Stretch

Place a pillow in the center of your bed. Lie on your left side with the pillows under your waist, your arms overhead, your right leg extended, and your left leg bent and resting on the bed, as shown in figure 8.15. If this is difficult, you can place a warm Fomentek bag or Mother Earth pillow beneath your waist. This is a completely passive stretch once you're in position, so just relax and enjoy it. Hold this position for 20 to 30 seconds and feel your body melt into the pillows. Stretch both sides even if you have pain on only one side.

Figure 8.15

Over a period of a few weeks, place additional pillows under your waist as you feel ready for a greater degree of stretch. To add the contract and relax component to this stretch, simply shorten your waist on the side you've been stretching by hiking up your hip toward your lowest ribs. Hold this contraction for at least 10 seconds, then exhale slowly as you completely relax the contraction and passively stretch again.

Advanced Side-Lying Stretch

This advanced stretch is effective for both the side of the waist and the hip. To stretch the right side, lie on a bed on your left side with your upper body and hips on the bed and your legs extending off the end, as shown in figure 8.16. Keep your right leg straight and your left hip and leg bent. Press your right leg downward toward the floor. Hold this stretch for at least 15 seconds. Repeat on the other side, even if you have pain on only one side. Repeat the stretch three times on each side, increasing the stretch slightly each time.

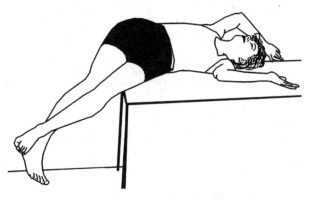

Figure 8.16

If this stretch is uncomfortable at first, try it while placing the foot on the side you're stretching on a stool or chair, as shown in figure 8.17. On the other hand, if you're able to tolerate a greater stretch, ask a partner to gently press down on the leg on the side being stretched.

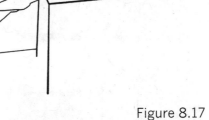

Figure 8.17

Stretching with a Fitness Ball

This stretch works best with a large fitness ball with a stability base. When you first try this, ask a friend to help make sure you don't fall off the ball. Start by placing the ball about 2 feet away from a wall and squatting next to the ball (on the side toward the wall), as shown in figure 8.18. Press your hip into the ball as you press your upper foot against the wall, as shown in figure 8.19. Next, lie over the ball on your side, supporting yourself with your lower arm, stretching the upper arm over your head, and spreading your feet apart, as shown in figure 8.20. Don't try this stretch at the beginning of self-care treatment; work your way up to it using the preceding stretches. To add the contract and relax component to this stretch, try to use your quadratus lumborum (and other muscles) to raise your torso up off the ball, as shown in figure 8.21.

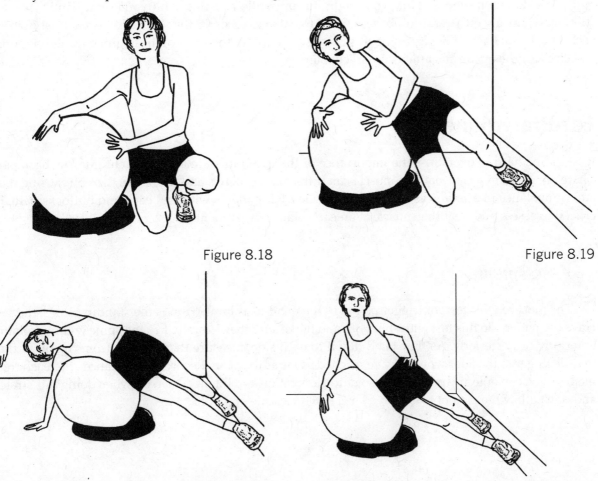

Figure 8.18

Figure 8.19

Figure 8.20

Figure 8.21

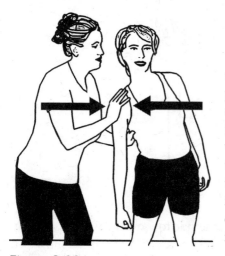

Figure 8.22

Contracting and Relaxing with a Partner

You'll need a partner to do this exercise. Stand with your feet shoulder width apart and slightly bend your knees. Have your partner place one hand on the side of your right shoulder and the other on your rib cage on the right, as shown in figure 8.22. Try to push your torso to the right with 30 percent of your strength while your partner resists. Push and hold for at least 15 seconds, then exhale and relax for 15 seconds. Repeat this exercise at least twice on each side. Each time, try to push a little harder, but hold for a slightly shorter time. This exercise is very satisfying, especially when performed after compression and stretching. Try to do it once or twice a day if you can find a partner.

Contracting and Relaxing Without a Partner

Stand with your feet shoulder distance apart. Place the palm of your right hand on your right hip and press down on the hip. Hike your right hip up while resisting with your right hand. This will contract your right quadratus lumborum. Hold for 10 to 15 seconds, then relax. Repeat at least twice on each side. If you have difficulty doing this exercise at first, try the some of the beginner range of motion exercises for the quadratus lumborum in chapter 16.

For Practitioners

It would be hard to overstress the importance of the quadratus lumborum in chronic low back pain. There are so many ways that this muscle can influence the pelvis and the spine, thereby causing muscular imbalance in as many as forty other muscles. For patients with low back and buttocks pain, it's crucial to assess and treat this muscle at an early stage of treatment.

Assessment

The most reliable test for trigger points in the quadratus lumborum is the standing side bend test. Have the patient do this test with shoes off, and make sure they laterally flex the spine without rotating anteriorly or posteriorly. As they bend down to each side, measure the distance from the tip of their middle finger to the floor when they've reached as far as they can. Record this distance after each treatment so you can note any progress. Also note the location and intensity of pain when doing this stretch, and don't allow the patient to exceed a level of 6 on a scale of 0 to 10.

Underlying Perpetuating Factors

We've found that the quadratus lumborum can be difficult to treat successfully if its trigger points stem from a long-standing structural imbalance, such as a small hemipelvis, leg length inequality, or short upper arm length. Treating the muscle without identifying and correcting for these conditions will provide temporary relief at best, so it's critical to test for these conditions and correct them when found. (See Mechanical Factors, in chapter 17, for details on structural imbalances.)

Treatment Techniques

Use of the Side-Lying Position

The side-lying position, as shown in figure 8.15, above, allows you to treat the quadratus lumborum on the stretch, yielding much better results. We recommend using a body support system on the treatment table. (Refer back to figure 2.1 to see the setup for this.) Patients are often surprised at how quickly their pain eases when this muscle is treated bilaterally on the stretch. We encourage our patients to replicate this stretch with pillows on their bed before going to sleep and upon awakening.

When treating the quadratus lumborum in this position, consider using a warm Fomentek bag under the waist and neck. In early stages of treatment, keep the stretch moderate, then increase the intensity as the patient is able to tolerate it. With severe activation of the quadratus lumborum, patients may be in too much pain to allow much stretching at first.

Beginning Treatment

For early stages of treatment, separate the two pieces of the body support system so the patient can place their arm and shoulder in the space between when lying on their side, as shown in figure 8.23. If you don't have a body support system, begin with the patient lying on their left side with a pillow under the head and neck and another pillow under the waist.

Press into the area of the quadratus lumborum and feel for taut bands, which can sometimes seem almost like a knife edge from the iliac crest upward to the lower ribs. Apply compression on these taut bands while directing the patient to lift the upper leg anteriorly while extending the upper body posteriorly as you treat the more anterior fibers of the muscle, as shown in figure 8.24. Palpate the superficial abdominal oblique muscles to determine if they also have trigger points, and treat them first if they do. Then have the patient roll the torso slightly anterior and

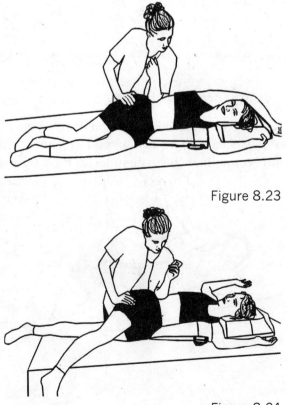

Figure 8.23

Figure 8.24

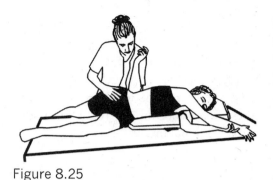

Figure 8.25

bring the thigh and leg posterior, as shown in figure 8.25, and treat the posterior portion of the muscle. Repeat this treatment on the opposite side, even if there are no trigger points on that side.

Intermediate Treatment

Fold the body support system on itself (doubling it up) and place a warm Fomentek bag on top of it, as shown in figure 8.26. If you don't have a body support system, use extra pillows to achieve a greater side-lying stretch. Have the patient assume a side-lying position over the body support system, as shown in figure 8.27, and treat as described above. Again, treat bilaterally, even if trigger points are present on only one side.

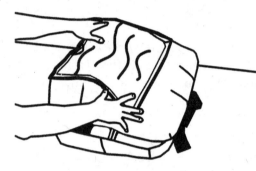

Figure 8.26

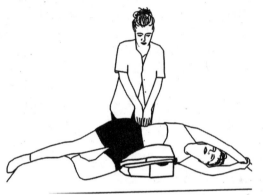

Figure 8.27

Advanced Treatment

To give the quadratus lumborum an even more acute stretch, have the patient move to the end of the table, with a body support system or pillows to support their head. To treat the left quadratus lumborum, have the patient lie on their right side with the right hip and knee flexed. The left leg is straight and hanging off the treatment table. This places the quadratus lumborum, gluteus medius, and gluteus minimus in an acute stretch. Try using a warm Fomentek bag or Mother Earth Pillow over the area being treated, as shown in figure 8.28. If the muscles are tight, heating the area is essential for the patient's comfort and relaxation; just treat right through the heat source. Compress both the anterior and posterior segments of the quadratus lumborum, and treat bilaterally as described above.

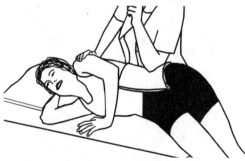

Figure 8.28

Spray and Stretch

Start by reviewing all the positions for side-lying treatment of the quadratus lumborum, above. Prior to employing spray and stretch treatment, make sure you have heat sources, such as warm Fomentek bags or Mother Earth Pillows, on hand. Position the patient as shown in figure 8.29. Holding the spray can at an acute angle, as shown in the figure, spray from the side from about 18 inches away, moving slowly—only about 4 inches per second. Spray along the lines shown in figure 8.29 and in the direction of the arrows, from superior to inferior, or over the trigger points in the

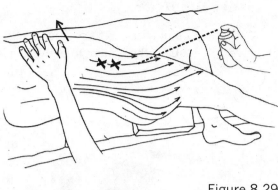

Figure 8.29

quadratus lumborum, and then over the referred pain pattern in the abdomen, groin, hip, buttocks, and sacrum. Afterward, apply heat while the patient is still in a stretched side-lying position.

Next, place the patient in the beginning, intermediate, or advanced side-lying position, as described above, and spray all the fibers of the quadratus lumborum. After completing the spray and stretch treatment, treat the entire sprayed area with heat for at least 5 minutes. Then turn the patient on the opposite side and repeat the entire spray and stretch procedure on the other side.

You can also apply the spray with the patient seated and stretching the quadratus lumborum or with the patient standing and stretching the quadratus lumborum with their arm extended overhead. Whatever treatment position you use, finish with the range of motion exercises for the quadratus lumborum in chapter 16.

Active Abduction

With the patient lying on their side, apply compression on the quadratus lumborum and instruct the patient to lift the thigh and leg while you provide gentle resistance against the knee, as shown in figure 8.30. The quadratus lumborum will contract as it works to stabilize the spine and pelvis as the leg abducts. Hold the resistance for 15 seconds, then have the patient exhale and relax as you slowly press farther into the quadratus lumborum. Variations of this resistance can be done with the torso rotated slightly anterior and the pelvis, thigh, and leg rotated posterior, and then reversing this position. Remember to do this on both sides, even if there's pain on only one side.

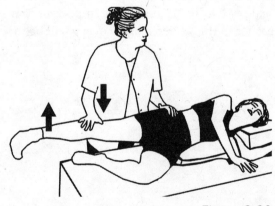

Figure 8.30

Active Hip Hiker

With the patient lying on their side, gently grasp the ankle and leg and pull downward, as shown in figure 8.31. Instruct the patient to perform a hip-hiking motion, attempting to raise the pelvis toward

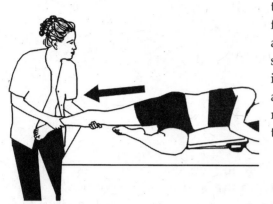

the rib cage, using 30 percent of their strength and holding for at least 15 seconds. Then instruct the patient to exhale and fully relax, then gradually drop the leg into a greater stretch off the back of the table behind the body, as shown in figure 8.25, above. Then have the patient do another active hip hike, and this time gradually drop the leg anteriorly off the table, as in figure 8.24, above. Do this at least twice on each side.

Figure 8.31

Summary

After treatment, notice if the patient's quadratus lumborum is softer than before and if compression is less painful. Next, have them stand, and check the symmetry of the pelvis, sacrum, spine, and scapulas. Repeat the standing side bend test and measure and note your findings. Keep notes on the level of compression the patient can tolerate during treatment, and also their level of discomfort on a scale of 0 to 10. It's especially important to instruct patients in a home self-care program, as described earlier in this chapter, as recovery will be much faster if they perform daily self-care treatment.

Chapter 9

Gluteus Maximus

In the good old days, the offices of the partners of the Morgan Bank in New York were situated on the main banking floor. In 1900 those bankers didn't sit at their desks, they stood at them. Given the time, a combination of factors probably motivated them to do so. There was respect for physical work because that's what most people did for a living; perhaps it seemed too much like leisure to be seen sitting while working. And, of course, business got done faster if conducted while standing. But perhaps they also knew something we've lost track of: Too much sitting is bad for your health!

Sitting comes in for much criticism in this book—because day in, day out we see the sad consequences of too much of it. The gluteus maximus muscle deserves much of the credit for humans being considered a "higher species." After all, it's largely due to the evolution of the gluteal muscles that we have the ability to stand erect, freeing our hands for other tasks.

But our modern society, with all of its computers, TVs, video games, desk work, and long commutes, has brought us down into a sitting position from elementary school through to our senior years. After millennia of hunting and gathering, our gluteal muscles are paying the price for this transformation into a sitting species, which is occurring too rapidly from an evolutionary point of view.

The gluteus maximus bears the bulk of the punishment from sitting all the time. It, more than any other, is the muscle we sit on. So if you have chronic trigger points in the gluteal muscles, you might follow the lead of those bankers a hundred years ago: Buy a desk at which you can stand instead of sit!

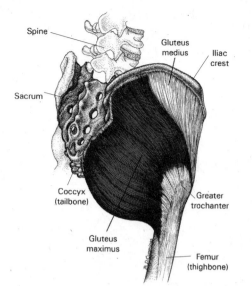

Figure 9.1

Where Is the Gluteus Maximus and What Does It Do?

The gluteus maximus is the largest of the muscles in the buttocks, and by weight, it's about twice as heavy as the other two gluteal muscles combined. It performs a good deal of the work involved in moving the thigh at the hip. As shown in figure 9.1, the muscle is attached to the side of the coccyx, part of the outer edge of the sacrum, and the back of the crest of the hip bone. Some of its muscle fibers also blend in with the tendinous mass of the superficial paraspinal muscles at the base of the spine, and with the fascia covering the gluteus medius. At the other end, some of the muscle becomes blended into the strong band of fascia that runs down the outside of the thigh, and it attaches on the outside of the thigh bone.

Always Stretched Is No Good

Unlike most of the other muscles involved in low back pain, the gluteus maximus gets into trouble not because it's chronically short, but because it's chronically stretched. Prolonged sitting without standing or movement puts these muscles in their most extended position. So when we ask you to stretch this muscle, it would be more accurate to say we want you to put the muscle through its full range of motion, from shortened to fully stretched, so it can work effectively through that full range. Movement through the full range of motion provides the best conditioning and overall health for our muscles.

The gluteus maximus plays a large part in stabilizing the body during walking and standing. A few million years ago, our forebears had more of a tail than we do now, and we still have very small vestigial muscles for that tail near the coccyx. In fact, in a very small percentage of the population these tiny "tail-wagging" muscles can be more developed and may actually contain trigger points that refer pain to the region of the coccyx. But this condition is so rare that we won't discuss it further.

Functions of the Gluteus Maximus

This workhorse muscle does several important jobs:

- It's a powerful extender of the thigh during activities such as jumping, running, climbing, and rising from a seated position.

- When we stand still, the gluteus maximus helps us maintain our upright posture.

- It assists in rotating the hip outward.

- During walking, the gluteus maximus helps maintain the body's position over the front foot.

- The gluteus maximus also works with some of the paraspinal muscles and the hamstrings to extend the trunk. In this movement, they help us come back to an upright posture from a bent-over position.

It's interesting that the gluteus maximus doesn't work hard during many common physical activities, such as walking. It more often comes into play as a stabilizer and a controlling muscle, such as when we bend forward and need to limit the extent of bending. In fact, when the gluteus maximus muscle is surgically removed on one side, it doesn't prevent the person from walking with a fairly normal gait. This shows how important the other gluteal muscles and the hamstrings are in walking.

Gluteus Maximus Pain Referral Patterns

The gluteus maximus contains three common trigger point regions, as shown in figure 9.2. The first is located in the upper part of the muscle next to the sacrum, as shown in figure 9.2A. The second is in the middle of the lower portion of the muscle along the border of the ischial tuberosities (the sit bones), as shown in figure 9.2B. The third is very near and just a bit below the tailbone, as shown in figure 9.2C. Figure 9.2D shows a composite of these three areas, along with the underlying anatomy.

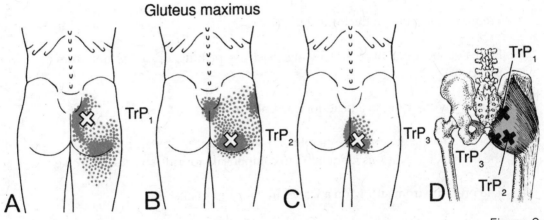

Gluteus maximus

Figure 9.2

While we're concerned with all three regions, in our experience the second region is the most common location for trigger points in the gluteus maximus. Trigger points here cause a sensation of pain in and around the sacrum and across the whole upper buttocks area. These trigger points are located very near the sit bones, and when we sit on them, the referred pain can be almost unbearable; it may feel as if you're sitting on a nail pressing into the sit bones. A doughnut-shaped cushion is sometimes prescribed to relieve this pain. If you have one, place the hole under the affected sit bone, as it's the pressure on this area that causes trigger points in the gluteus maximus and the resulting referred pain. This may help relieve the tension and pressure on the second trigger point region.

Trigger points in the third region, near the coccyx, cause a great deal of discomfort around the tailbone when sitting, even though the tailbone never touches the chair. Trigger points in the gluteal muscles are often found on one side, rather than both, because many people tend to place more weight on one side when sitting, sleeping, or driving (Travell and Simons 1992).

What Aggravates the Gluteus Maximus?

Several activities can cause or exacerbate tension and trigger points in the gluteus maximus:

- Walking uphill or up stairs, especially when bent over

- Sitting for long periods slumped backward onto your buttocks and tailbone, which can activate trigger points in the second and third region

- Sudden overload, as with a slip or near fall

- Falling on the gluteus maximus or a direct blow to the muscle

- Sleeping on your side in a fetal position, with your knees pulled up

- Sleeping flat on your back with your legs straight

- Frequent injections in the buttocks

- Repeated bending over and lifting, such as picking up an infant from the floor or a playpen

- Habitually standing in a head-forward posture

- Morton's foot syndrome (see chapter 17), which causes tightening of the horizontal fibers of the gluteus maximus as it attempts to compensate for this structural problem

- The pressure from sitting on a wallet in your hip pocket

- Vigorous upward kicking, as when swimming the crawl stroke and doing the flutter kick—especially in cold water

Do I Have Trigger Points in My Gluteus Maximus?

Several symptoms point particularly to trigger points in the gluteus maximus:

- Pain and tenderness throughout the buttocks after sitting, especially pain around the sit bones, or a feeling like you're sitting on a knife

- Pain deep in the buttocks or in and around the tailbone

- Difficulty walking uphill or up stairs, especially when bent forward

- Squirming in your seat during prolonged sitting in an attempt to avoid local tenderness and referred pain

- Difficulty finding a comfortable chair

- Difficulty bringing your knee to your chest while lying flat on your back

- Difficulty contracting the gluteus maximus when swimming the crawl, especially in cold water

- Pain in the buttocks when partially reclining with knees straight

- A tendency to walk with toes pointed outward

Simple Tests

Three simple tests can help you determine whether you may have gluteus maximus trigger points: the knee to armpit test, the seated toe touch in a chair, and the seated toe touch on the floor. However, because all the gluteal muscles share tasks to some degree (along with other muscles in the hip and pelvic region), the tests below can't point conclusively to one specific muscle as containing trigger points. Fortunately, it's easy to treat all the gluteal muscles as a group, as described in chapter 12.

Knee to Armpit Test

While you can do the knee to armpit test by yourself, it's better to have a friend assist you. While lying on your back on a carpeted floor or yoga mat, bring one leg up toward your chest. Grasp your leg behind your thigh, not over your knee, and pull your thigh up and as far toward your opposite armpit as you can. Keep your knee and abdominal muscles relaxed. If you can bring your knee quite close to your chest, as shown in figure 9.3, it's unlikely that trigger points are present in your gluteus maximus. If you can go only as far as shown in figure 9.4, you may have trigger points in your gluteus maximus.

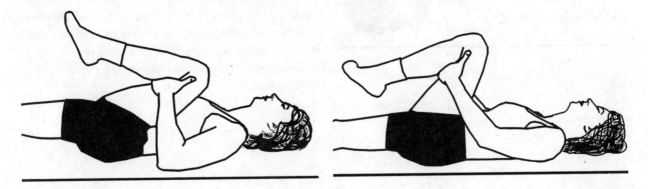

Figure 9.3   Figure 9.4

If you feel pain in your buttocks when you pull your thigh toward the opposite armpit, this is a definite indicator of trigger points.

If a friend is assisting you, have them press your thigh into your chest rather than you doing the pulling. This allows you to more completely relax your gluteus maximus, abdominal, and iliopsoas muscles, which otherwise could restrict your range of motion. Note that this test also measures the length of the hamstrings and the ability of the iliopsoas to shorten. So an inability to bring your knee to your shoulder can be an indicator of trigger points in any of these three muscles: gluteus maximus, hamstrings, or iliopsoas.

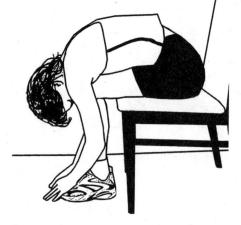

Figure 9.5

Seated Toe Touch in a Chair

To more directly isolate the gluteus maximus, sit in a stable and comfortable chair, lean forward, and reach toward your toes, as shown in figure 9.5. If you're able to place your hands flat on the floor, you don't have trigger points in your gluteus maximus. (Even if you have extra belly fat, you should still be able to reach the floor with the tips of your fingers.) If you can't, you probably have trigger points in your gluteus maximus.

Seated Toe Touch on the Floor

Do this test while sitting on a carpeted floor or yoga mat. Extend your right leg in front of you and bend your left leg at the knee, allowing it to rotate to the side a bit. Bend forward at the hip without lifting your thigh off the floor and, with both hands, reach as far as you can toward the toes of your right foot, as shown in figure 9.6. If you're forty or younger, you should be able to reach at least to your toes; if you can't, you probably have trigger points in your gluteus maximus. Give yourself an extra inch of gap for every decade over forty, and see how close you can get. Pain in the buttocks while doing this test is also an indication of trigger points in the gluteus maximus. Note that this also tests the paraspinals and hamstrings, so if you can't pass this test, you should consult chapters 6 and 13 to determine whether you have trigger points in those muscles.

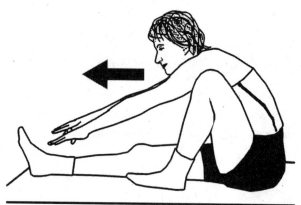

Figure 9.6

Helpful Hints for Eliminating Trigger Points in the Gluteus Maximus

Although your muscles can't talk, they can still tell you what to do and not do—if you'll just pay attention to them. If it's very painful to sit, that could be your gluteal muscles saying, "I've had enough! Get up and get some exercise!" Here are a few simple things you can do to help eliminate trigger points in the gluteus maximus:

- If you must sit for long periods, change your seated posture from time to time so you distribute your weight to different areas of the buttocks. Limit your sitting to 20 minutes, then get up and walk around for a few minutes, varying your movements as much as possible, particularly your hip movements, and then resume your work. Set a timer to go off every 20 minutes to remind you to stand up and move around. In chapter 16, you'll find range of motion exercises that target the gluteals. Do one or more of those exercises during every break.

- If you sleep on your side, keep your legs extended and in alignment with your hips and shoulders, rather than tucked up with your knees bent. Also try placing a pillow between your lower legs from the knees to the feet. If you sleep on your back, place an overstuffed pillow under your knees. (See chapter 17 for more on sleep positions.)

- When lifting anything heavy, keep your torso upright and your knees bent, rather than bending forward from the waist.

- Sit on a coccyx cushion with the hole centered under one or the other buttock, not under the tailbone, even though the pain may be there.

- Limit climbing and walking uphill as much as possible until you've effectively treated your gluteal muscles.

- Avoid leaning over a work surface for an extended period.

- Stop carrying your wallet in your hip pocket, and definitely don't sit on it.

- Try sitting on a seat wedge or a large exercise ball. By using different seating options, you can vary your posture, even if only a little, to avoid sustained pressure on the same spots all the time.

- Note that when treating the gluteus maximus, it's important to also assess and treat the hamstrings (see chapter 13).

In our experience, it's common to have trigger points in the gluteal muscles primarily on one side or the other. However, it's also common to have trigger points in several if not all the gluteal muscles on one side. Fortunately, it's easy to treat all these muscles at the same time. For specifics on treatment, see chapter 12, Combined Buttocks Treatment.

Chapter 10

Gluteus Medius and Gluteus Minimus

The two smaller gluteal muscles are the gluteus medius and gluteus minimus. Travell and Simons called the gluteus medius the "lumbago" or "low back pain muscle" and the gluteus minimus the "sciatica muscle." Their nicknames reflect the fact that these muscles often account for much of the pain associated with these common diagnoses.

Trigger points in the gluteal muscles and the iliopsoas, as well as muscular entrapment of some of the superficial nerves that serve these muscles, can cause pain, numbness, tingling, and tightness all the way from the buttocks to the toes. Interestingly, this cluster of symptoms is quite similar to those in the fairly new diagnosis of restless legs syndrome. If you've been given this label, it may be worth your while to try self-care for the gluteal muscles before resorting to the various prescription drugs being offered for restless legs syndrome.

Where Are the Gluteus Medius and Gluteus Minimus and What Do They Do?

The gluteal muscles are located on either side of the sacrum and provide most of the muscular tissue in your buttocks or hips. Most of this muscle group consists of the gluteus maximus, covered in the preceding chapter. The gluteus maximus is usually more than twice the size of the gluteus medius, and the gluteus medius is more than twice the size of the gluteus minimus. Think of the gluteus medius and minimus as broad, thin layers of tissue, each covered by its bigger "brother." The gluteus maximus partially covers the posterior of the gluteus medius, and the gluteus minimus is completely covered by the gluteus medius. Together, these two smaller muscles help stabilize the pelvis while walking, running, or standing on one leg, and both help lift the thigh toward the chest (the medius more than the minimus).

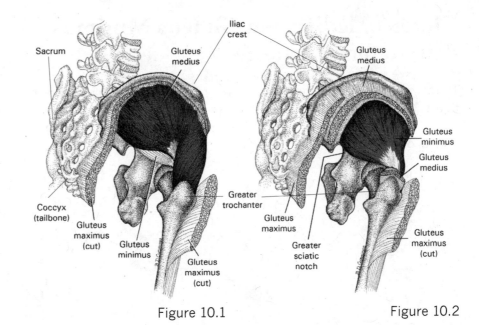

Figure 10.1   Figure 10.2

The gluteus medius, shown in figure 10.1, attaches to most of the outer surface of the pelvis and runs down to the top of the femur. Underneath the gluteus medius's tendinous attachment to the femur lies the trochanteric bursa, a sac that cushions the interface between the tendon and the bone. Many of our patients who have pain in the hip at that location have been told that they have bursitis of the hip. However, when we eliminate trigger points in the gluteus medius and restore full range of motion through active self-care by the patient, the "bursitis" often disappears.

The superficial fibers of the gluteus medius closest to the front of the body actually twist and run in a different direction than those toward the back. This coincides with the different functions of the fiber sections. The twisted section of fibers toward the front assists in turning the leg inward, and the posterior fibers assist in turning the leg outward. The gluteus medius as a whole is a major player in lifting the thigh outward.

The gluteus minimus, shown in figure 10.2, is the smallest and deepest of the three gluteal muscles. It attaches to the pelvis along the outer surface of the hip bone about an inch or more below its crest. From there it travels downward to the front surface of the upper femur, where it attaches by its tendon. Just like the gluteus medius, the gluteus minimus contributes to lifting the thigh outward, with the front portion of the muscle helping to turn the leg in, and the back portion of the muscle helping to turn the leg out, Travell and Simons 1992).

Gluteus Medius and Gluteus Minimus Pain Referral Patterns

Trigger points in the gluteus medius refer pain to the buttocks and upper outer thigh, as shown in figure 10.3. In most cases, if you experience pain in the buttocks and upper thighs, this is a reliable indicator of trigger points in the gluteus medius. This low back and buttock pain is often referred to as lumbago.

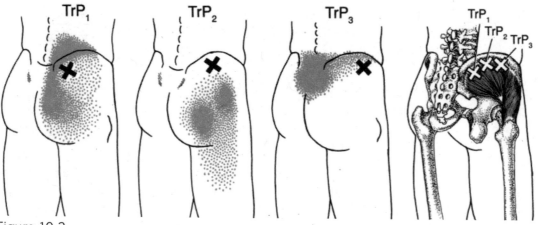

Figure 10.3

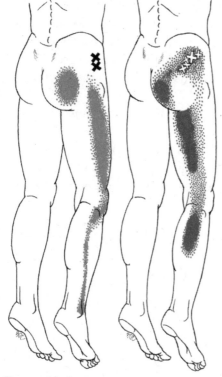

Figure 10.4

In the gluteus minimus, there are two distinct trigger point regions. The first is located in the front part of the muscle. Trigger points here refer pain to the buttock and straight down the outside of the thigh to the knee, calf, or ankle (see figure 10.4 [left]). Trigger points in the back part of the muscle refer pain to the hip, lower buttock, the back of the thigh, and the back of the calf, as shown in figure 10.4 (right).

Sciatic pain is often described as pain running down the outside of the thigh and lower leg, often down as far as the ankle. Sometimes it can be at the back and side of the buttocks. The pain is more often felt on one side or the other, although it can occur on both sides. Sciatica is usually experienced as being deep in the hip, often severe, persistent, and accompanied by tenderness throughout the thigh, leg, and ankle. It can wake you up or prevent you from sleeping. People complaining of this type of pain are often diagnosed with sciatica, implying compression of the sciatic nerve. However, in our clinical experience, when treatment of the gluteus minimus relieves this pain, it confirms that there wasn't any impingement of the nerve—merely the symptoms associated with such compression. When this happens, it's better to use the term "pseudo-sciatica," meaning that the symptoms are present, but the actual nerve impingement is not (Travell and Simons 1992).

What Aggravates the Gluteus Medius and Gluteus Minimus?

Many things can contribute to trigger points in the gluteus medius and gluteus minimus, with seated posture being a frequent cause of problems. (As you work with the various chapters in this book, you'll no doubt notice that this is a recurring refrain.) In this case, problems arise due to asymmetries and chronic contraction. Fortunately, two common causes of asymmetry are relatively easily to deal with, once you know about them: the rich man's problem and the driver's problem.

The rich man's problem. Believe it or not, sitting on a thick wallet (or even a thin one) can compress the muscle fibers of the gluteus medius and minimus, causing trigger points and pain in the buttocks, the thigh, and down the leg. Because it's more common to carry the wallet in the right hip pocket, this generally causes problems on the right side.

The driver's problem. If you drive a great deal, your right leg probably remains in a fixed position for long periods, especially if you don't have cruise control. This is a common cause of trigger points in the gluteus minimus and, less commonly, the gluteus medius. Obviously, this causes problems primarily on the right side, although if you assume an abnormal seated position when driving it may cause other problems as well.

Here are some other factors that can contribute to trigger points in the gluteus medius and gluteus minimus. For more information on many of these issues, see Mechanical Factors, in chapter 17:

- Leg length inequality, which causes your gluteal muscles to tighten on one side to compensate

- Morton's foot syndrome

- Dysfunction of the sacroiliac joint, where the sacrum joins the pelvis

- Standing still for long periods, especially with your weight on one leg or with your feet close together, as the leg and hip muscles tend to contract more to maintain balance

- Sleeping on your side in the fetal position or without any support for the top leg

- Sleeping on your back with your feet splayed out under the weight of a heavy blanket

- Repetitive overuse of the gluteal muscles during sports such as running, tennis, or golf, and sports injuries or falls

- Injections in the buttocks

Do Trigger Points in the Gluteus Medius and Gluteus Minimus Muscles Affect Posture?

Postural imbalance can be either a cause or an effect of trigger points in the gluteal muscles. As noted above, leg length inequality and Morton's foot syndrome are common causes of gluteal trigger points. A chronic head-forward posture can also cause trigger points in the gluteal muscles. But sometimes it works the other way around.

Severe pain caused by gluteal trigger points can lead to limping or an unusual walking posture in an attempt to moderate the severity of low back or hip and leg pain. This kind of compensation can lead to a cascade of other pain problems resulting from abnormal gait or posture.

Do I Have Trigger Points in My Gluteus Medius or Gluteus Minimus?

The location and severity of pain is a good indicator of whether the gluteal muscles are involved and can also help identify which of the muscles is the culprit. Look at the pain referral patterns shown in figures 10.3 and 10.4. If your pain looks like any of the pain referral patterns in figure 10.3, focusing primarily on the center of the buttocks or in and around the sacrum, that points to trigger points in the gluteus medius. If the pain is in your buttocks and also runs down the side or back of your leg, as shown in figure 10.4, that points to either the gluteus minimus or the piriformis. When the pain in your leg extends into the lower leg and calf, you're more likely to find trigger points in the gluteus minimus.

A number of common problems can indicate active trigger points in either the gluteus medius or the gluteus minimus. Trigger points in either of these muscles often cause pain that's so persistent and severe it interferes with sleeping and walking, and you may have to use a cane while walking. It's common to be unable to find any position that relieves the pain. Trigger points in either muscle can also prevent you from raising your leg out to the side, make it hard to stand on one leg, or give you a feeling of weakness in the hips while walking. Because of the persistence and severity of pain caused by trigger points in these two muscles and the inability to find any position that gives relief, many people resort to painkillers or even surgery.

Simple Tests

Five simple tests can help you determine whether you may have trigger points in the gluteus medius or gluteus minimus. However, because all the gluteal muscles share tasks to some degree (often along with other muscles in the hip and pelvic region), the tests below can't point conclusively to one specific muscle as containing trigger points. As you'll see below, many of these tests may also indicate trigger points in the piriformis (the third group of gluteal muscles, covered in chapter 11). Fortunately, it's easy to treat all the gluteal muscles as a group, as described in chapter 12.

Turning Your Feet In and Out

This test is exceedingly simple. Stand up and look at your feet. Do you normally stand or walk with your feet in a turned-out position? This may indicate chronic tightness and shortening in your gluteus medius, gluteus minimus, and piriformis, as well some small muscles deep in the pelvis. First, see if you can turn your feet inward. To do this, you must rotate your thigh bone inward. This movement stretches the piriformis and other muscles whose job is to turn the hip, leg, and foot outward. If turning your feet in is difficult, or if you experience pain when you do so, you probably have trigger points in the gluteus medius and minimus and possibly other muscles as well.

Next, try to turn your feet out. If this is difficult or painful, you may have trigger points in your gluteus medius, gluteus minimus, or piriformis, or other hip muscles.

Bonnet's Sign Test

To test for restriction in the left gluteus medius and gluteus minimus, as well as the piriformis, start by lying on your back on a carpeted floor or yoga mat. Keep your right leg straight, bend your left knee, and place your left foot flat next to the outside of your right calf. Slide your left foot upward as far as you comfortably can, as shown in figure 10.5, keeping both buttocks and your foot flat on the floor as you do this. If your left heel comes up as high as the top of your right knee and you don't experience any pain, you probably don't have trigger points in the left gluteus medius or minimus. If you can't get your foot that high or it's painful to do this test, that indicates trigger points in either the gluteus medius, gluteus minimus, or piriformis, or other muscles deep in the pelvis. Do this test for both sides.

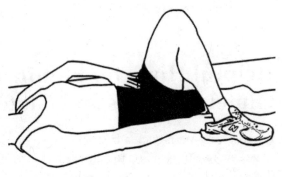

Figure 10.5

Pace Abduction Test

Sit in a chair and have a friend place their hands on the outside of both of your knees. Ask them to hold your knees in position, then try to push your knees outward against their hands. If this is painful or you can't push out on either side, it may indicate trigger points in the gluteus medius, gluteus minimus, or piriformis.

Standing Leg Swing Out

While holding on to a sturdy chair or other support, swing one leg outward two or three times while standing on the other leg. Then turn and test the other side. Positive indicators for trigger points in the gluteus medius or minimus include the following:

- Pain during this movement

- Difficulty doing the movement

- Cramping or near cramping of the hip muscles

- Inability to stand on either leg by itself

- Uneven or jerky movement during the leg swing

Knee Crossing Test

To perform this test, simply cross your left leg over the right while sitting erect in a chair, and notice the position of your left knee. If it completely crosses your right knee, there's no limitation of your range of motion and you probably don't have trigger points. If your left knee won't cross completely over your right knee, this indicates trigger points in the left gluteus minimus. If you can get only your ankle or part of your left calf over your right knee, you probably have trigger points in both the gluteus minimus and the piriformis. Test both legs and note any restriction of movement on either side. It's common to find a problem on only one side.

Helpful Hints for Eliminating Trigger Points in the Gluteus Medius and Gluteus Minimus

Because driving is such a frequent cause of problems in the gluteus medius and gluteus minimus, we have several suggestions to help with this problem. When possible, use cruise control so your right leg doesn't have to hold a fixed position. If extensive driving is unavoidable and you have chronic buttock pain, notice when and where you have pain and look for trigger points in the muscles that refer pain to that area. Take frequent breaks from driving to stretch those muscles and use them in their normal range of motion. Also, try to move your right leg and change your driving position as often as every 10 minutes. You can also try using a tennis ball under the right buttock to see if it relieves the pain. If you have a long stop-and-go commute, as millions of people do these days, experiment with different seating positions on different days, or use a seat wedge on some days to vary your position.

Here are a few more simple things you can do to help alleviate trigger points in the gluteus medius and gluteus minimus:

- Use seating variations such as Fomentek bags or seat wedges.

- If you must stand for a long periods of time, don't stand on one leg. Also, keep your feet at least a foot apart and shift your weight from one leg to the other periodically.

- Stop carrying a wallet in your hip pocket.

- Don't wear high heels, or wear them only occasionally.

- Sleep on your side with a pillow between your knees.

- If you tend to overuse your gluteal muscles during sports activities, do self-care beforehand and afterward.

- If you have a chronic head-forward posture, treat and stretch the muscles in the upper back and neck to correct for this. This isn't an easy postural imbalance to correct, and doing so will take time even if you work at it. However, in some cases it's a major cause of chronic trigger points in the gluteal muscles.

- Have a trained practitioner check you for leg length inequality and Morton's foot syndrome. (See Mechanical Factors, in chapter 17, for more on these conditions and how to remedy them.)

In our experience, it's common to have trigger points in the gluteal muscles primarily on one side or the other. However, it's also common to have trigger points in several if not all the gluteal muscles on one side. Fortunately, it's easy to treat all these muscles at the same time. For specifics on treatment, see chapter 12, Combined Buttocks Treatment.

Chapter 11

Piriformis

If you've ever done the twist, you were doing a range of motion exercise for the piriformis muscle. This muscle lies deep in the buttocks underneath the gluteus maximus and, together with other muscles, helps keep the thigh bone in the hip socket. Trigger points in the piriformis can cause pain in the low back, buttocks, sacrum, and hips. This muscle generally doesn't act alone in causing low back and hip pain. We often find that it's one of several muscles in the buttocks region containing trigger points. Since we sit so much, it's hardly surprising that the buttocks muscles are a major factor in pain problems.

Dr. Travell called the piriformis the "double devil" because it can cause two distinct pain problems: First, active trigger points in the piriformis can refer pain into the buttocks and down the back of the leg. Second, although the piriformis is a small muscle, it passes through a rather narrow space. If the muscle becomes enlarged due to chronic shortening, it can potentially entrap blood vessels or nerves, including the sciatic nerve, that also pass through that same small space. This problem is sometimes referred to as piriformis syndrome. Compression of the sciatic nerve can cause pain, numbness, and tingling in the buttocks, thigh, and lower leg. In some cases, the pain associated with chronic taut bands in the piriformis is so persistent and severe that surgery is performed to relieve the pressure.

Because there are several possible causes of the pain and other symptoms associated with piriformis syndrome, a physician's diagnosis is necessary to determine an appropriate course of treatment. Malignancies, infections, arthritis, herniated disks, spinal stenosis, displacement of the sacroiliac joint (where the sacrum joins the pelvis), or structural imbalances can all cause or exacerbate the symptoms of piriformis syndrome. Interestingly, there can be significant variations in the shape of the piriformis and its spatial relationship to the sciatic nerve. In fact, in about 20 percent of people, the piriformis is split and the sciatic nerve actually passes through the main bulk of the muscle (Klein 2006). Given these anatomical variations, it is easy to see how chronic taut bands of muscle fiber in the piriformis (or other nearby muscles) could cause sciatic nerve impingement.

With these symptoms and conditions, the first priority must be to determine whether there are non-muscular causes of the pain and dysfunction. If you can safely rule them out, our clinical experience suggests that most people suffering from these symptoms can be successfully treated by the methods described in this book. At any rate, it certainly seems sensible to try the self-care protocols described in chapter 12 before resorting to surgery.

Where Is the Piriformis and What Does It Do?

The piriformis is located under the gluteus maximus and gluteus medius muscles, deep in the upper part of the buttocks as shown in figure 11.1. The piriformis is the primary muscle in a group of six called the *short lateral rotators*. At the inner end, the piriformis is attached to the inside surface of the sacrum. Laterally, it's attached to the head of the thighbone by a tendon it shares with other deep hip muscles. It runs across the buttocks (though with a slight downward angle from the sacrum to the thighbone), rather than up and down the body like most of the other muscles we discuss in this book.

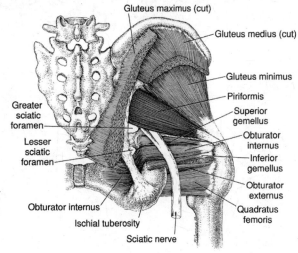

Figure 11.1

The other five short lateral rotators are located just below the piriformis and also run from side to side, as can be seen in figure 11.1. These muscles act primarily to turn your thigh and leg in or out. The piriformis, on the other hand, has several actions, and the position of the thigh and leg affects the way this muscle functions:

- It turns the thigh outward when the leg is straight or extended back.

- It stabilizes the hip joint and helps hold the femur in the hip socket.

- While standing and during weight-bearing activities, the piriformis prevents or checks too-rapid inward rotation of the thigh.

- When seated in an upright position or when on all fours, the piriformis helps move the leg out to the side.

- When the thigh is pressed to the chest, the piriformis can bring the knee inward.

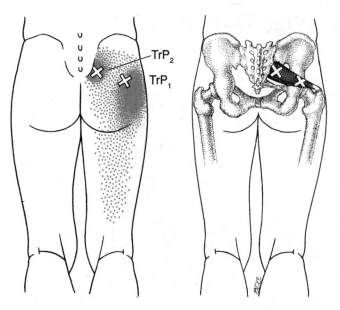

Figure 11.2

Piriformis Pain Referral Patterns

Trigger points (shown by X's) in either the inner or the middle part of the piriformis refer pain primarily to the area of the sacrum, the entire buttock, and most of the way down the back of the thigh, as shown in figure 11.2. As mentioned, a chronically contracted piriformis can entrap the sciatic nerve and possibly others, leading to various symptoms associated with sciatica. These include pain and numbness in the low back, groin, perineum, buttocks, hip, leg, and even foot, as well as sharp pain in the rectum during defecation. A sensation of pain running down the thigh and leg can also be caused by referred pain from trigger points in the gluteus minimus, in which case it is more properly referred to as "pseudo-sciatica."

What Aggravates the Piriformis?

There are several distinct ways that trigger points become activated in the piriformis muscle:

- Sudden overloading of the muscle, for example, during lifting or lowering a heavy object. Such overloading can also occur during a fall, catching yourself to prevent a fall, or an impact trauma, such as a car accident.

- Repetitive overuse of the muscle, perhaps the best example being outward leg lifts from an all-fours position (sometimes known as "fire hydrants"). Repetitive overuse can also occur among distance runners.

- Prolonged contraction of the muscle. Driving a car without stopping for long periods is a frequent cause of trigger point activation. When you have your right foot on the gas pedal without interruption for hours at a time, which usually involves prolonged contraction of the piriformis and other muscles on the right side, is it any wonder that you might develop problems with these muscles?

- Sitting with one foot underneath you or cross-legged.

- Walking with your toes out. This can be due to Morton's foot syndrome (see chapter 17), which causes chronic shortening of the piriformis and other lateral rotators.

- Underuse caused by sitting for long periods without moving the lateral rotators through their normal range of motion.

Other, less common causes of trigger points in the piriformis include infections (including pelvic inflammatory disease), arthritis in the hip joint, and other structural problems such as unequal leg length or a small hemipelvis.

Do I Have Trigger Points in My Piriformis?

If walking is painful or you tend to drag one leg or limp, that may indicate trigger points in the piriformis. If you tend to squirm or shift your weight from side to side when seated, that's another possible indicator of trigger points.

Four simple tests can help you determine whether you may have trigger points in the piriformis: the knee crossing test, turning your feet in and out, Bonnet's sign test, and the Pace abduction test (the latter is considered one of the most reliable tests for trigger points in the piriformis). All four are described in detail in chapter 10. Be aware that because all the gluteal muscles share tasks to some degree (often along with other muscles in the hip and pelvic region), these tests can't point conclusively to one specific muscle as containing trigger points. Fortunately, it's easy to treat all the gluteal muscles as a group, as described in chapter 12.

Helpful Hints for Eliminating Trigger Points in the Piriformis

The exercises in chapter 16 will help restore normal range of motion in the piriformis. Even 5 to 10 minutes of focused movement and stretching a day can help a chronically taut muscle return to normal function. In addition, here are a few simple things you can do during normal daily activities to help restore circulation and improve range of motion in the piriformis:

- Change your seated position frequently, or stand occasionally as an alternative.

- Avoid sitting cross-legged or on your feet. This is very important.

- When driving for a long time, periodically take a break to get out and walk around, and use cruise control whenever possible.

- Use a warm Fomentek bag under your bottom when seated.

- Avoid carrying your wallet in your hip pocket.

- In general, when you walk, keep your feet pointing straight forward. If your feet generally turn out, take action to remedy this.

- As a therapeutic exercise, walk for a short distance with your toes in, and then with your toes out. Repeat this sequence several times daily.

- When walking, roll through your entire foot, from heel to toe, and be sure to push off with your toes, which will encourage movement of the piriformis. In order to walk through your foot, you must wear flexible shoes.

In our experience, it's common to have trigger points in the gluteal muscles primarily on one side or the other. However, it's also common to have trigger points in several if not all the gluteal muscles on that side. Fortunately, it's easy to treat all these muscles at the same time. In fact, to treat trigger points in the piriformis, you have to compress other, more superficial buttocks muscles on your way to the piriformis anyway. For treatment of all these muscles, see chapter 12, Combined Buttocks Treatment.

Chapter 12

Combined Buttocks Treatment

While each of the buttock muscles has a different primary function, they're all located in the same part of the body and are layered over one another, so they can, for the most part, be treated in the same positions and using the same techniques. In fact, when you treat the deeper gluteal muscles, you often treat the overlying muscles by default. For these reasons, we've combined treatment of all these muscles into a single chapter. The muscles covered in this chapter are the gluteus maximus, gluteus medius, gluteus minimus, and piriformis, as well as deep rotators lower down in the buttocks. For more information on these muscles, their pain referral patterns, diagnostic tests and tips on what to do (and not do) to keep them healthy, see chapters 9, 10, and 11. Also, please note that it's important to assess and treat the hamstrings (see chapter 13) when treating the gluteus maximus.

Many of the self-care techniques described below call for using various balls, rollers, and other tools because it can be difficult to reach behind you to compress the muscles in the buttocks region. For guidance on self-compression, look at figures 12.1 through 12.4 on the following page. The smaller X's represent all areas where you should apply compression. The larger X's represent the most likely places to find trigger points. It's important that you treat all the areas marked with small X's, applying more sustained compression to any areas that are firmer or more painful. If you feel discomfort when you compress specific areas, this confirms that trigger points are located there and need treatment. Try to relax as much as possible as you apply compression in these spots, and reduce the amount of compressive force, if need be, by using a different tool, modifying your body position, or applying less body weight or force. When the pain of self-compression decreases noticeably, you can apply more compression or do it in a stretched position.

Here are some general pointers for all treatment techniques described in this chapter:

- Warm the area prior to treatment, especially when your symptoms are severe.

- When sitting or lying on the floor for any form of self-care (compression, stretching, range of motion exercises), a carpeted surface is ideal; alternatively, you can use an exercise mat.

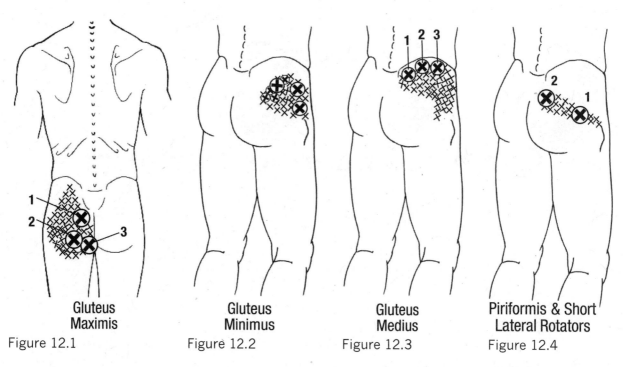

Gluteus Maximis	Gluteus Minimus	Gluteus Medius	Piriformis & Short Lateral Rotators
Figure 12.1	Figure 12.2	Figure 12.3	Figure 12.4

- Treat both sides, even if you appear to have trigger points on only one side. The two sides are synergists and frequently work together to do the same job, so trigger points often develop on both sides. Or after trigger points develop on one side, the other side may overwork to compensate, causing new trigger points to develop. This is particularly important in treating the buttocks muscles.

- Refer to the muscle illustrations and compress all areas indicated by X's. The larger X's represent likely spots for trigger points, but the entire muscle requires treatment.

- Never exceed a pain level of 6 on a scale of 0 to 10.

- When applying compression, sustain the compression for up to 30 seconds and repeat at least two or three times, or until there's a noticeable decrease in pain and increase in range of motion.

- Gradually increase the amount of compression as you feel the muscle softening and relaxing. Be aware of how the tissues respond to treatment.

- When stretching, hold the position for two to three normal breaths.

- When a stretch is repeated several times on both sides, alternate sides with each repetition.

- After treatment and stretching, do the range of motion exercises for the gluteal muscles and piriformis in chapter 16.

Warm-Up

You can warm the entire buttocks region by sitting on a warm Fomentek bag or Mother Earth Pillow for 5 to 10 minutes. If you have time, a better warm-up for the buttocks is to soak in a warm tub for up to half an hour before applying compression. You can also use gentle range of motion exercise (see chapter 16) as a warm-up before compression.

Compression

Beginner Level

You can use a Mother Earth Pillow as a source of heat and mild compression at the same time. Fold a heated pillow to provide a firm, flat area, place it on the floor, and sit on it. Allow your body weight to press your buttocks onto the pillow, as shown in figure 12.5. Place most of your weight on the buttock you're treating, breathe, and relax. Move slowly from one spot to another until you've treated all areas of the buttock. Change the angle of your hips and lean sideways onto your elbow to compress a little higher or lower on the outside of your buttock, as shown in figure 12.6. You can achieve more intense compression by crossing one leg over the other, as shown in figure 12.7. You can also shift your weight and position to apply greater compression on the inner or outer portions of the buttock. Even if you have pain only on one side, treat both buttocks. This beginner compression can also be done seated in bed or in a firm chair or lying down.

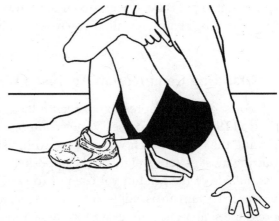

Figure 12.5

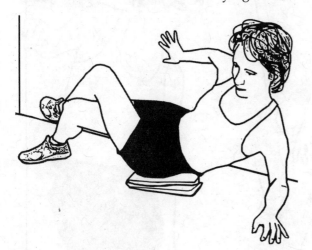

Figure 12.6

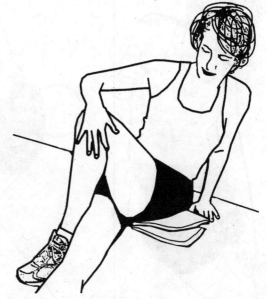

Figure 12.7

You can also use an Orbit Massager to treat the superficial area of the buttocks. Try lying on your side and bending the knee up toward the chest to stretch the gluteal muscles while using the Orbit Massager, as shown in figure 12.8.

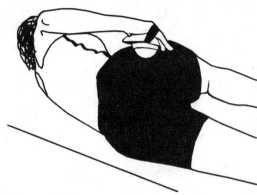

Intermediate Level

As you achieve greater mobility and less pain in your buttocks with compression as described above, you can start using intermediate techniques, which provide more

Figure 12.8

concentrated pressure. If you're confident in your balance, use various compression tools while standing or leaning against a wall. If you're unstable on your feet, start in bed on a soft ball.

Standing Compression Against a Wall

For standing compression of the buttocks, use a warm, folded Mother Earth Pillow, as shown in figure 12.9. You can also use a 7-inch compression therapy ball against a wall, as shown in figure 12.10, placing the ball between you and the wall, using your legs to press your buttocks onto the ball, and putting most of your weight on the opposite foot. Move the ball slowly around the entire buttock, from the outside of the head of your femur to your sacrum, looking for painful spots. If you're especially tender in certain areas, adjust the pressure so it's tolerable. Be sure to turn your body sideways to compress the side of the buttock and the area around your thighbone at the hip socket, as shown in figure 12.11.

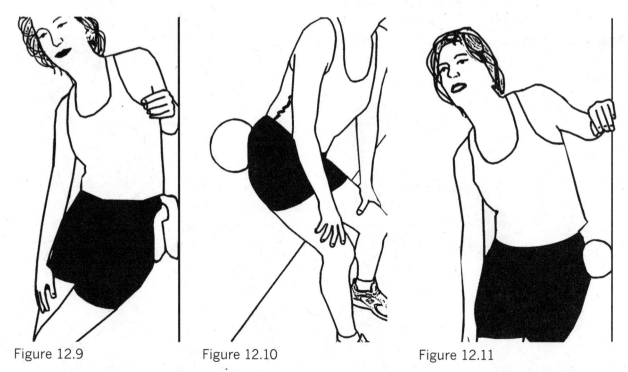

Figure 12.9   Figure 12.10   Figure 12.11

Pain and tenderness during compression indicates that you're pressing on the right spot. Sustain the pressure on these spots for at least two full breaths, then gradually relax and release the pressure by shifting your weight slightly away from the wall. Then move your hip over the ball so the compression occurs an inch or so away from the previous spot. A total of a dozen different compressions spaced about an inch apart will cover most of the area to be treated. In each spot, use as much compression as you can without exceeding a level of 6 on a pain scale of 0 to 10.

Compression While Lying Down

If your gluteal muscles are very tender but you're able to tolerate firm compression, try treatment while lying in bed. (As mentioned above, this is also useful if you aren't steady on your feet.) In the center of your bed, set up some pillows or a folded blanket to provide support for your upper body, then lie on your side over the support and place a 7-inch compression therapy ball under your buttock, as shown in figure 12.12. Use your upper leg to help you balance on top of the ball and also to help you move over the ball onto different locations on your buttocks. The relative softness of the bed will determine the amount of compression you feel. Try to keep your spine in a neutral position during compression. You can also turn onto your back, as shown in figure 12.13, and use the same leg to help move you over the ball. If this is too painful at first, simply deflate the ball until it provides a therapeutic level of compression without excessive pain.

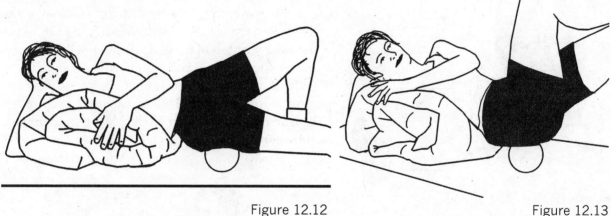

Figure 12.12   Figure 12.13

Advanced Level

After a couple of weeks, you probably won't be able to reach a pain level of 6 out of 10 with a 7-inch compression therapy ball. At this point, you're ready for more advanced compression, as described below.

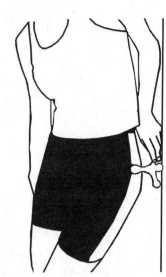

Figure 12.14

Compression While Standing

For more concentrated compression while standing, you can use a 5-inch compression therapy ball, a Jacknobber, or a Backnobber. You can even use a tennis ball or racquetball inside a stocking or long sock. Because of their smaller size, these tools will apply more concentrated pressure on any given area, so don't be overly aggressive at first. Gradually lean more of your body weight into the tool, as shown in figure 12.14, and move around the buttocks until you find painful or tender spots.

Compression on the Floor

Many self-care tools can be used for advanced treatment of the buttocks muscles while sitting or lying on the floor, including a 5-inch compression therapy ball, a foam roller, a tennis ball, or a Backnobber. You might find it easiest to start doing compression on the floor using a foam roller, as shown in figure 12.15. This provides excellent compression over a broader area and is more stable than a ball. Remember to apply compression over the entire buttock from bottom to top, and also lean to the side, as shown in figure 12.16, to get at the outer portions of the gluteal muscles. When using a compression therapy ball, you may need to deflate it slightly to reduce the pressure if compression is too painful at first. If it's difficult to balance on top of the ball, use a couch or chair to provide additional support, as shown in figure 12.17.

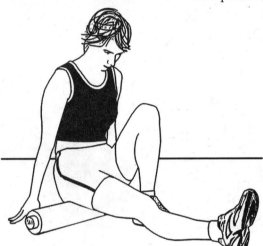

Figure 12.15

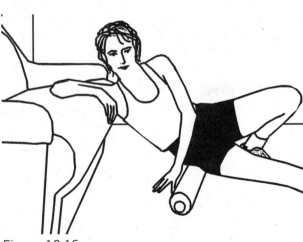

Figure 12.16

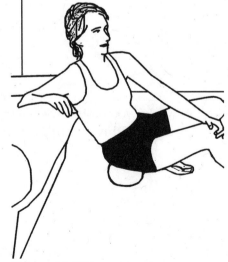

Figure 12.17

If you find this method of treatment too painful, go back to doing the compression on your bed, using pillows or a folded blanket to support your upper body, as before. You may even want to drape a warm Fomentek bag over a foam roller, as shown in figure 12.18. The key is to listen to your body and adjust what you're doing so that you keep making progress without excessive pain.

The Backnobber is the most precise tool for compression while lying on the floor. Position the tool as shown in figures 12.19 and 12.20 and press upward on the upper part of the S curve, allowing the tool to do most of the work. Note that the positions shown in these figures stretch the gluteal muscles gently by crossing one leg over the other. If that's too much first, just keep both feet flat on the ground.

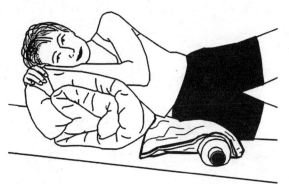

Figure 12.18

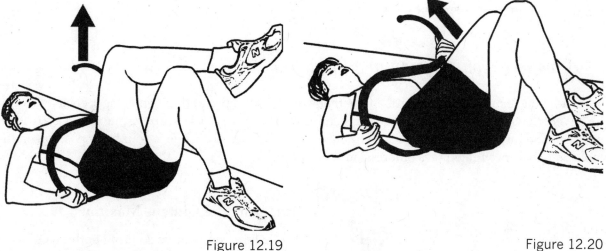

Figure 12.19   Figure 12.20

If you work with a 7-inch compression therapy ball, you can inflate the ball to achieve greater compression as the muscles become less painful. Place the ball under your buttock, then move your buttock slowly over the ball until you've covered the entire buttock and hip area. Adjust your body position as needed, as described for the intermediate level. Treatment while lying on your side, as shown in figure 12.21, is particularly good for treating the gluteus medius, the gluteus minimus, and the *tensor fasciae latae* (a small muscle just below the widest part of the hip and close to the greater trochanter). The position shown in figure 12.22 is more effective for the gluteus maximus, the short lateral rotators in the hip, and the hamstring attachments on the sit bones.

Be careful to control the amount of pressure you place on the ball, especially at first. Don't simply place all of your body weight on the ball right off; gradually roll onto the ball and increase the amount of weight on it very slowly until you reach a discomfort level of about 6 out of 10.

When you've reduced your initial tenderness and sensitivity in the gluteal region with the 7-inch ball on the floor, you can begin to use the 5-inch treatment ball. It might take a month or more before you reach that point. Repeat the same process as before. Use your hands and arms to maintain stability and adjust the compressive level on the ball as you roll your buttock over it. You can also use even

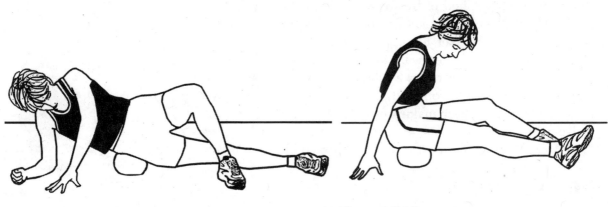

Figure 12.21

Figure 12.22

smaller or harder treatment balls, such as a softball, baseball, tennis ball, or racquetball. Use these balls just as you would a larger compression therapy ball, but monitor the compressive force carefully as it will be much more spot-specific with these smaller tools.

Advanced Compression in a Stretched Position

Once you've mastered the treatment methods described above and they no longer elicit a discomfort level of 6 out of 10, you're ready to apply compression to the buttocks with the muscles in a stretched position. You can use any of the tools mentioned above. What will change is your body position on the tool and how concentrated the compression is on specific areas.

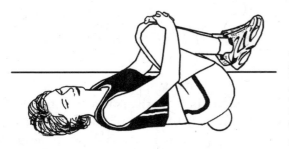

Targeting the Gluteus Maximus

While lying on your back, bring both knees up to your chest and place a firm treatment ball under your buttock, as shown in figure 12.23. Use your arms to pull your thighs up to your chest and keep your abdominals relaxed. Allow the weight of your legs and pelvis to compress the gluteal muscles into the ball. After three relaxed breaths, reach down and move the ball an inch or two and repeat this sequence all over the gluteal muscles, leaning your body and legs to one side to compress the sides of the muscles.

Figure 12.23

For another stretched position to target the gluteus maximus, sit on the floor with your legs straight out in front of you, place a ball or foam roller under your buttocks, and reach forward and grasp your socks or calves, as shown in figure 12.24. Hold this stretch for 20 seconds as you apply compression, then relax, reposition the ball, and repeat until you've treated as much of the buttocks as you can reach in this position. Initially, you may find it easier to start with just one leg extended and using a foam roller, as shown in figure 12.15, above.

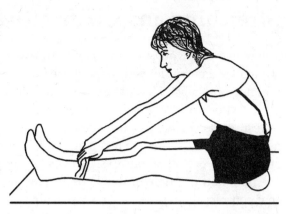

Figure 12.24

Targeting the Gluteus Medius, Gluteus Minimus, and Piriformis

To treat the right side, balance on a compression therapy ball in a seated position and place your

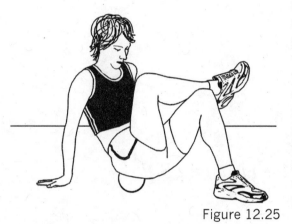

Figure 12.25

right leg and foot across your left thigh, as shown in figure 12.25. Try to bring the knee of your right leg closer to your chest to maximize the stretch. You might want to use pillows or a folded blanket to help support your body weight as you apply the compression. Place as much of your weight onto the ball as you can comfortably tolerate. This will compress the stretched piriformis, as well as the gluteal muscles. You can also place a warm Fomentek bag on top of the ball and apply compression with heat. Move your buttocks over the ball, as described above, to compress all the areas indicated with X's.

Compression Summary

As you continue treatment over several weeks, you should notice gradual improvement in the tightness, tenderness, and painful spots in your buttocks. If you had been experiencing numbness and tingling, those symptoms should also be noticeably reduced. The key is patience. As you begin to achieve a pain-free state, keep in mind that you can best maintain that state by doing a little self-care every day.

Stretching and Contracting

Below, we give you many different stretches for the buttocks. We've indicated which muscles each stretch targets, but let your experience be your guide. Those that cause more discomfort are the ones you need the most. Find the exercises that work best for you and begin doing them gently at first. The object is not pain, but mobility. The discomfort is just a sign you're asking a partially shut-down muscle to resume its normal function. Find the sequence that works best for you and do it several times a day as long as you continue to feel pain. Work your way up from the beginning exercises to the advanced stage over a period of four to six weeks (or more) as you gain flexibility.

As noted throughout this book, stretching is more effective if done in conjunction with exercises that contract the muscle. This is particularly important for the buttocks muscles, as most of us spend many hours a day sitting, which puts these muscles in a stretched position. For this reason, most of the stretches below include contraction and relaxation phases. In this chapter, the stretches are divided into five different positions:

1.   Stretching while lying on the floor or a bed

2.   Stretches while sitting on the floor or a bed

3.   Stretches while sitting in a chair

4.   Stretches while standing

5.   Stretch with the legs off the edge of a bed

Stretch and Contract While Lying on the Floor or a Bed

Beginner Level: Single Knee to Armpit

(Gluteus maximus and hamstrings)

While lying on your back, bring your right leg up toward your chest. Grasp your leg behind your thigh, not over your knee. Keeping your abdominal muscles relaxed, use both arms to pull your knee toward your armpit, as shown in figure 12.26. When you can pull the leg no farther, hold for two slow breaths. Next hold your thigh firmly while you push away with 30 percent of your strength, as if trying to return your thigh to the floor, for 15 seconds. This contracts the muscles. While remaining in this position, with your knee to your chest, relax your gluteal muscles. Do this stretch and contract three times on each side, trying for a slightly greater stretch each time. Do this exercise on both sides even if you have pain only on one side. For a variation on this exercise, pull your thigh toward the opposite armpit.

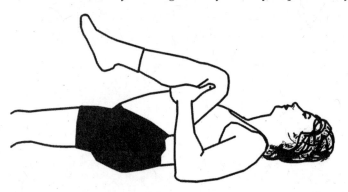

Figure 12.26

Beginner Level: Double Knee to Chest

(Gluteus maximus and hamstrings)

Lie on your back and slowly pull both knees up toward your chest, as shown in figure 12.27, keeping your abs relaxed. Hold for two deep breaths, then lower your legs and relax. After this gluteal stretch, it's a good idea to do a gentle abdominal stretch (see chapter 7).

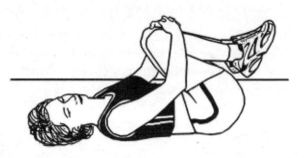

Figure 12.27

Intermediate Level: Leg Crossover Stretch and Contraction

(Piriformis)

If you have very tight hip rotator muscles, this stretch will be difficult. Just do the best you can,

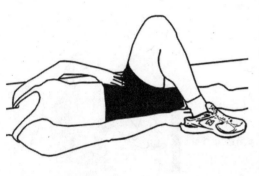

Figure 12.28

and don't exceed a pain level of 6. While lying on your back, cross your left leg over your right and place your left foot flat on the floor as close to your right knee as you can, as shown in figure 12.28. Reach down and grasp your ankle or the back of your shoe, then pull the foot toward your hip, keeping both buttocks and your foot flat on the floor. Breathe slowly and deeply and stay relaxed. To add the contraction and relaxation components, try to straighten your left leg while maintaining a firm grip on your shoe or ankle. Hold this contraction for 15 seconds, then exhale as you stop resisting, and fully relax. After another 20 seconds, slowly pull your left foot a bit farther toward your right hip. Do this twice on each side.

Intermediate Level: Knee Crossover Stretch and Contraction

(Piriformis)

While lying on your back, cross your left leg over your right leg as in the previous stretch, then use your right hand to pull your left knee and thigh over and downward, as shown in figure 12.29. Breathe and stay relaxed, especially in your abdomen and hips. To add contraction and relaxation, you'll need a friend to provide resistance. Have your friend push against the outside of your left knee as you press against them with 30 percent of your strength. Hold the resistance for 15 seconds, then exhale slowly as you relax. Do this stretch three times on each side, trying to pull the thigh a bit farther across your chest each time.

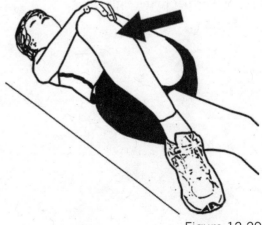

Figure 12.29

Advanced Level: Leg Fall-Over Stretch

(Gluteus medius, gluteus minimus, and piriformis)

While lying on your back, cross your left leg over your right knee, then relax and allow your legs to gently fall over to the left, as shown in figure 12.30. Relax into the stretch for three deep breaths, then repeat on the other side. The first few times you do this stretch, use a large pillow to control the extent of the stretch and how far your lower back twists. Over time, you can decrease the height of the pillow and allow your legs to fall farther and farther. When your thigh reaches the pillow, relax and note where you feel the stretch. If you feel it more in your low back, you need to treat your paraspinal muscles (see chapter 6). If you feel the stretch mostly in your left hip, your paraspinals are in good shape. Perform this stretch three times on each side.

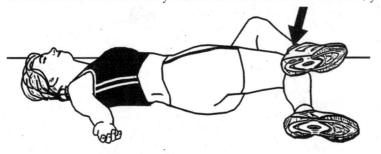

Figure 12.30

Intermediate Level: Strap-Assisted Stretch and Contract

(Gluteus medius and gluteus minimus)

While lying on your back, place a loop of a stretching strap around the arch of your left foot (or use a dog leash). Cross your right leg over your left and place your right foot flat on the floor next to your left knee. Use the strap to pull your left leg to the right, as shown in figure 12.31, keeping the leg extended and resting on the floor. You should feel the stretch in the outside of your left gluteal muscles. Hold the stretch for 20 seconds, then relax. Repeat for the other leg.

To add contraction, hold the strap firmly and pull the leg to the left against the resistance of the strap for 15 seconds, using 30 percent of your strength. Exhale, relax completely, and repeat this sequence three times for each leg, each time relaxing fully and then pulling the leg a bit farther to the right.

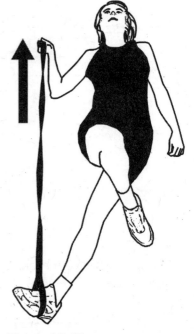

Figure 12.31

Stretches and Contractions While Sitting on the Floor or a Bed

Beginner Level: Hugging Your Knee

(Gluteus maximus, gluteus medius, gluteus minimus, and piriformis)

Sit on the floor and cross your right leg over the left, placing your right foot flat on the floor next to your left knee. While keeping your abs relaxed, hug your right thigh with your left arm and pull it close to your chest, as shown in figure 12.32. Hold this stretch for 10 seconds, then relax. To add contraction after the stretch, maintain a firm grasp on the knee and try to rotate the knee out to the right with 30 percent of your strength, using your gluteal muscles to do this. Hold the contraction for 15 seconds, then exhale slowly and relax. After 20 seconds, pull the right thigh a little closer to your chest than before. Perform this sequence three times on each side.

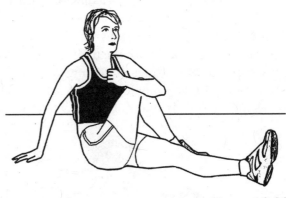

Figure 12.32

Beginner Level: Butterfly Stretch and Contraction

(Piriformis and adductors)

Sit on the floor with your knees bent. If you're sufficiently limber, place the bottoms of your feet flat against each other, as shown in figure 12.33. Spread your knees apart in a relaxed position and hold for two or three relaxed breaths. Note whether you feel any discomfort or restriction as your knees drop out toward the floor. If you feel discomfort in your groin, your *adductors* (the muscles that bring your thighs together) are tight. If you feel discomfort in the outside of your hips, then your piriformis muscles can't fully relax when they're shortened.

To add contraction, press your legs apart with 30 percent of your strength while resisting with your hands or arms on the outside of your knees, as indicated by the arrows in figure 12.33. Hold this position for 10 seconds, then relax completely as you exhale. Next, place your elbows on the inside of your knees, then attempt to bring your knees together against this resistance, again using 30 percent of your strength. Hold the contraction for 10 seconds, then relax. Repeat this exercise twice more, each time using just a bit more strength to resist the pressure of your hands. Don't apply more resistance than you can comfortably tolerate when pressing either in or out on your knees.

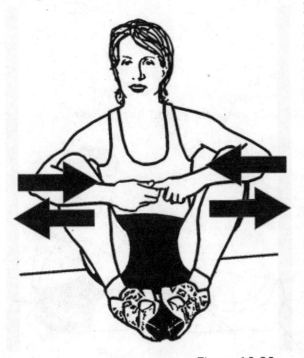

Figure 12.33

Intermediate Level: Seated Single-Leg Toe Touch

(Gluteus maximus, hamstrings, lower leg muscles, and some paraspinals)

If the intermediate and advanced seated stretches with contraction are particularly painful, use a warm Fomentek bag or Mother Earth Pillow under your buttocks or thighs. Do this intermediate stretch with contraction twice a day for at least two weeks before progressing to the advanced level.

While seated on your bed or the floor, extend your right leg and bend your left knee, allowing it to fall out to the side a bit, as shown in figure 12.34. Stretch your torso down toward the toes of your right leg, reaching forward with the fingers of both hands and keeping your abs relaxed. Feel your gluteus maximus and hamstrings stretching as you reach toward your toes. Hold this stretch for at least 15 seconds, then relax completely. Switch legs and reach toward the toe of the other foot. Repeat three times for each leg. If you're able to reach only your knees at first, don't worry; the object isn't to reach a

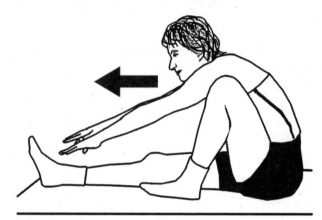

certain point, but to extend the stretch over time. Note the distance from your outstretched fingertips to your toes and use this information to monitor your progress over time.

To add the contraction component, grasp your right ankle or calf with one hand and pull your torso back against this resistance with 30 percent of your strength. Hold the contraction for 20 seconds, then relax for 15 seconds. Go through the entire sequence three times for each leg. Over time you can progress to grasping the leg with both hands, then eventually move on to the double-leg stretch described below.

Figure 12.34

Advanced Level: Double-Leg Toe Touch

(Gluteus maximus, hamstrings, lower leg muscles, and some paraspinals)

Sit with both legs extended in front of you. Relax your abs, exhale, and lean forward, grasping your calves or ankles with both hands, as shown in figure 12.35. Initially, you may find it difficult to get into this position; just reach as far down your legs as you can. Hold the stretch for two full breaths.

To add contraction, continue holding your legs, press your heels into the floor, and try to bring your back to an upright position using 30 percent of your strength. Hold this contraction for 15 seconds, then relax. Repeat this sequence at least three times, trying to stretch just a bit farther forward each time.

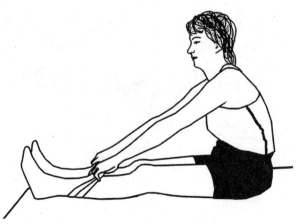

Figure 12.35

Stretch and Contract While Sitting in a Chair

These stretches and contractions are easy to do at home or at work. If you spend a lot of time in a seated position, do them as often as once an hour to prevent ill effects from constant sitting.

Beginner Level: Seated Knee Press

(Piriformis, gluteus minimus, gluteus medius)
Sit in a chair and place your hands on the outside of your knees. Using 30 percent of your strength, press your thighs outward while resisting with your hands. Hold for 10 seconds, then exhale and gradually relax. Next, make fists with both hands and place them end to end between your knees. Squeeze your knees together with 30 percent of your strength, hold for 10 seconds, then exhale and gradually relax. Repeat this sequence three times.

Beginner Level: Seated Leg Crossover Stretch

(Gluteus minimus, gluteus medius, piriformis)
While seated, cross your right leg over your left thigh and allow both thighs to rest against each other as shown in figure 12.36. Repeat three times on each side.

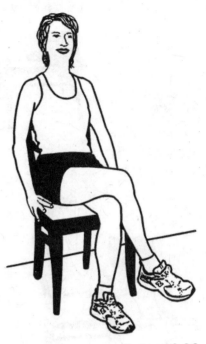

Figure 12.36

Beginner Level: Chair Stretch Sequence

(Rectus abdominis, gluteus maximus, iliopsoas, paraspinals, hamstrings, and soleus)
This sequence, which can be done in less than 5 minutes, takes each of the buttocks muscles through their full range of motion. If you have buttock pain, make this sequence part of your daily routine. All you need is a chair without armrests.

1. Sit on the chair and bend forward in your chair and rest your hands on the floor (or as close to the floor as you can get), as shown in figure 12.37, and hold for two relaxed breaths.

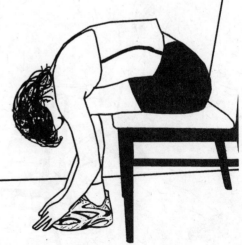

Figure 12.37

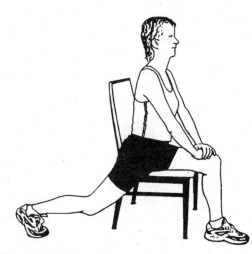

Figure 12.38

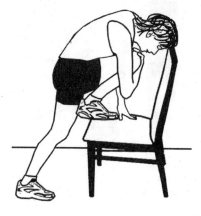

Figure 12.39

2. Scoot to the right side of the chair and stretch your right leg out to the back, placing your weight on your left buttock and keeping your torso upright, as shown in figure 12.38. Hold for two relaxed breaths.

3. Stand with your right foot on the chair, then bring your chest down to your knee, as shown in figure 12.39, keeping your abs relaxed. Hold for two relaxed breaths.

4. Place both feet on the floor, hold on to the back of the chair, and extend your right leg backward, as shown in figure 12.40, contracting the buttocks. Keep your body upright and allow your pelvis to sink toward the floor. Hold for two relaxed breaths.

5. Raise the same leg up behind you, as shown in figure 12.41, and hold this position for 10 seconds.

Repeat the entire sequence on the other side.

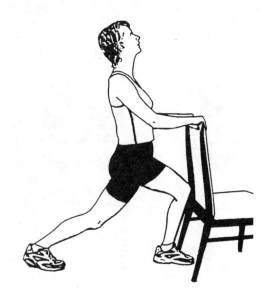

Figure 12.40

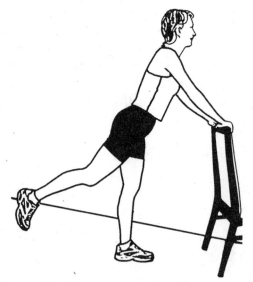

Figure 12.41

Intermediate Level: Seated Figure 4 Stretch

(Piriformis, gluteus minimus, gluteus medius)

Sit in a chair and cross your right leg over the left, placing your right ankle on your left thigh, as shown in figure 12.42. Note how close to horizontal you can get your right leg. If your knee is really high up or if you can't assume this position, you definitely have muscular restriction due to trigger points in your gluteal muscles. Don't worry; just keep trying to do this stretch as best you can. Over time you'll be able to bring the leg closer to a horizontal position.

To add contraction and relaxation, remain in the stretched position and place your right hand on the inside of your right thigh. Push gently downward with your right hand as you try to bring your thigh upward using 30 percent of your strength. Hold this contraction for 15 seconds. Relax, exhale, and then gently press your right leg farther downward (but not so far as to cause discomfort). Next, place your hands at the outside of the knee and press the right thigh downward against the resistance of your hands, again using 30 percent of your strength. Hold the resistance for 10 seconds. Exhale, gradually relax, and then attempt to hug the thigh to your chest, using your hands to pull the thigh upward, as shown in figure 12.43. Do this sequence three times on each side.

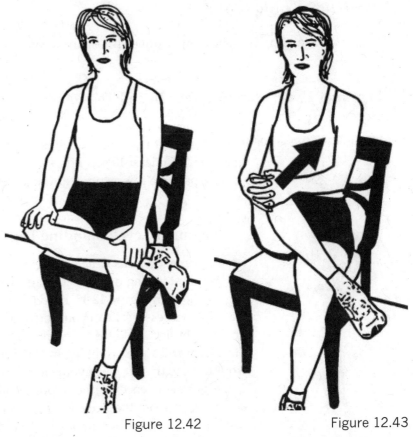

Figure 12.42   Figure 12.43

Intermediate Level: Seated Floor Touch

(Gluteus maximus, gluteus minimus, gluteus medius, piriformis, paraspinals)

Sit in a chair, cross one leg over the other, then bend down and try to touch the ground, as shown in figure 12.44. Do this exercise at least three times for each leg.

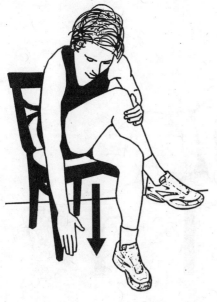

Figure 12.44

Stretches While Standing

These easy standing stretches can be done almost anywhere, anytime.

Beginner Level: Standing Toes In and Toes Out

(Piriformis, gluteus medius, and gluteus minimus)
For this gluteal stretch, just stand with your toes pointed inward and then outward. Hold each position for at least 10 seconds, and repeat at least three times. For chronic gluteal pain, do this as often as once every hour.

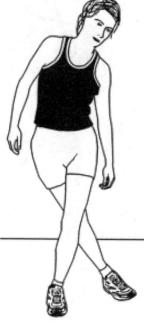

Beginner Level: Standing Leg Cross

(Piriformis, gluteus medius, and gluteus minimus)
While standing on your left leg, cross your right leg behind your left leg, as shown in figure 12.45. Hold on to a sturdy chair or other support for balance if necessary. Lean your torso to the left and push your right hip out to the right side. Hold for 10 seconds. This stretches the muscles of the right hip. Then cross your right leg in front of your left leg and once again lean your torso to the left, push your right hip outward, and hold for 10 seconds. Repeat the sequence on the opposite side. As you're able to do this with less pain, increase the stretch gradually by pushing the hip farther out and crossing the leg farther across, both behind and in front of the other leg. Repeat these stretches three times on each side.

Figure 12.45

Stretch with Legs Off the Edge of a Bed

Intermediate Level

(Gluteus medius and gluteus minimus)
Try this stretch before getting out of bed in the morning. If your pain is primarily on one side, lie on the opposite side with your hips at the edge of the bed and allow the upper leg to hang off the bed, as shown in figure 12.46. If this is too much of a stretch, you can support the foot on a footstool. Remain relaxed and hold this position for 20 seconds. Repeat on the other side. When you've done this three times for each leg, roll onto your stomach, drop both legs off the bed, place your feet on the floor, and get up.

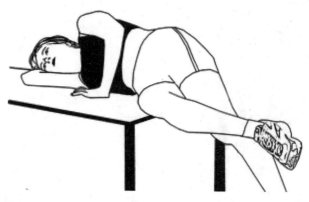

Figure 12.46

For Practitioners

When one of the gluteal muscles contains trigger points, the others usually become activated to some degree as well. Since these muscles are in such close proximity to each other, we often treat segments of more than one muscle during compression. To help determine which muscle you're treating at any particular time, you can ask the patient to perform the primary action of that particular muscle. Palpating the ensuing contraction of the muscle helps identify which muscle you are treating.

For example, in the side-lying position, abduction of the hip when flexed 90 degrees is the primary responsibility of the piriformis. Prone, knee-bent hip extension with slight lateral rotation is the primary responsibility of the gluteus maximus. And side-lying straight-leg abduction with a slight medial or lateral rotation will work the gluteus medius and gluteus minimus.

Also, please note that it's important to assess and treat the hamstrings (see chapter 13) when treating the gluteus maximus.

Additional Diagnostic Tests

The chapters on the individual buttocks muscles (chapters 9 through 11) include a variety of diagnostic tests for the buttocks muscles. Here are a few more you may find useful.

Coffee-Table Test

The coffee-table test assesses stretch range of motion in the piriformis, the gluteus medius, and the short lateral hip rotators (sometimes called the *gogos,* an acronym for superior **g**emellus, **o**bturator internus, inferior **g**emellus, and **o**bturator externus). Have the patient lie on their side, and stabilize their pelvis by pressing into their upper hip with one hand. Holding the ankle, raise the top leg and support it against your abdomen, as shown in figure 12.47, with the femur level with the greater trochanter. (In this position, you could balance a cup of coffee on it, hence the name of the test.) Next, while continuing to hold the patient's ankle, instruct the patient to drop their knee to the table, as shown in figure 12.48. If the knee won't drop all the way to the table, that's a positive indicator for trigger points

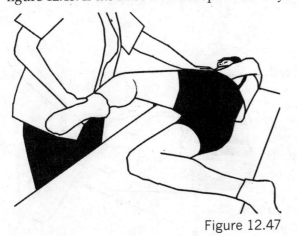

Figure 12.47

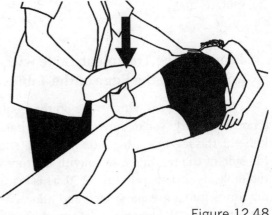

Figure 12.48

in one or more of the muscles mentioned above.

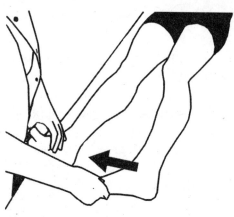

Figure 12.49

External Rotators Test

This tests the stretch range of motion of the piriformis, the gluteus medius and minimus, and the gogos. With the patient lying supine with legs extended, rotate the leg medially, as shown in figure 12.49, and measure the distance between the table and the big toe. The medial aspect of the foot should lie flat on the table. If the patient's knee rises off the table or if this causes pain, that indicates trigger points in one or more of the muscles listed.

Treatment Positions for the Gluteal Muscles

In general, treating the gluteal muscles on the stretch will yield better results than treating them in a neutral position. We generally treat in a neutral position only at the outset, and then for a short time only. For the gluteus maximus, hip flexion provides a good stretch. For the gluteus medius and minimus, adduction with internal or external rotation with the patient lying on their side will stretch most of the fibers. To effectively treat the piriformis, the hip needs to be flexed at least 90 degrees; some degree of adduction, internal rotation, or both will help maximize the stretch. Remember to treat the muscles on both sides, even if only one side has trigger points.

Prone on the Treatment Table with Hip Flexed

With the patient lying prone on the treatment table on a body support system, bring the hip and knee being treated into flexion. This will bring the knee up almost level with the patient's chest. This stretches the gluteus maximus and shortens the piriformis and other deep lateral rotators. With the patient in this position, you can use your elbow to press up and inward to the lowest trigger points in the gluteus maximus.

Prone on the Treatment Table with Hip Flexed and Leg Off the Edge of the Table

With the patient lying prone on the treatment table on a body support system, have the patient bend the hip and knee of the leg being treated. The knee should hang off the side of the treatment table with the foot remaining on the table, as shown in figure 12.50. This brings the gluteus maximus into a greater stretch and allows better access to the piriformis, the lower part of the gluteus maximus, and the gogos.

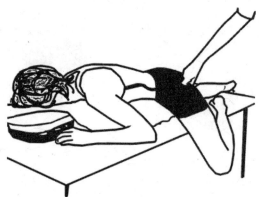

Figure 12.50

To add range of motion and treat the piriformis, gluteus medius, and gluteus minimus, adduct and abduct the leg while applying compression with your knuckles, as shown in figure 12.51. If you abduct the leg farther, you can use your elbow, as shown in figure 12.52.

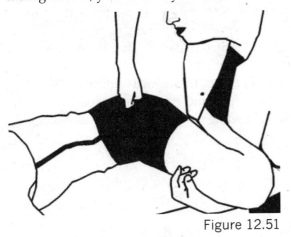

Figure 12.51

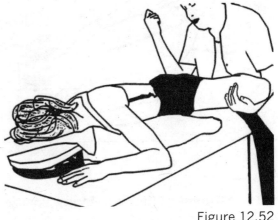

Figure 12.52

Treating Prone with Hip Extension

Treating the gluteal muscles while shortened can reveal taut bands of tissue that inhibit movement through the full range of motion. Active hip extension by the patient during treatment can help retrain the muscles.

To assess the gluteal muscles with the patient lying prone, ask the patient to bend their knee slightly. Holding the knee, laterally rotate the leg and raise it about a foot off the table, as shown in figure 12.53. If the gluteus maximus is working properly, it should feel evenly firm as you palpate it over its entire surface. Let the patient relax and return to the starting position. If trigger points are present, have the patient repeat this hip extension while you treat with active contraction and relaxation. Have the patient actively contract the muscle with 30 percent of their strength for 10 seconds. (The hamstrings will also be working during this contraction.) Then have the patient inhale and exhale while completely relaxing. Repeat this treatment until you notice a definite increase in range of motion and the patient reports reduced pain levels.

Place your knee on the treatment table and use it for stability and leverage. Place one arm under the thigh and raise it into extension as you hold down the hip with your other elbow or forearm, as shown in figure 12.54. This will also stretch the iliopsoas, the hip flexors, and the lumbar back. Don't exceed the patient's comfort level, and make sure the erector spinae and abs are relaxed in this position.

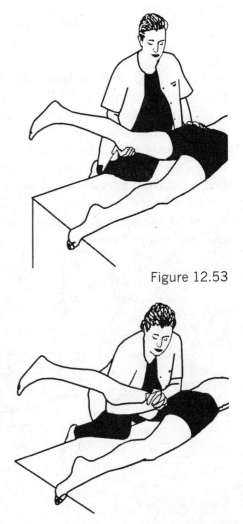

Figure 12.53

Figure 12.54

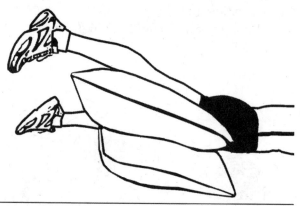

Let the patient's thigh rest on your thigh, or place a bolster under the leg, as shown in figure 12.55. With the muscle in this passive, shortened position, use your elbow to compress the gluteus maximus. Sometimes muscles with active trigger points will twitch while in a shortened position, or they may be unable to relax even though they aren't actively working. In such cases, warm Fomentek bags on the abs and the gluteal muscles can help relax them while you're treating in this position.

Figure 12.55

Treatment in the Side-Lying Position

Since many patients with back pain experience pain or discomfort while lying on their side, we recommend using a body support system when treating in this position, along with Fomentek bags slightly filled with warm water under the lower hip and thigh. Have extra warm Fomentek bags on hand in case you want to apply compression to the top leg through heat.

Treating the gluteus medius in the side-lying position: Have the patient lie on their side with the painful hip up. If this position is too painful, place a pillow between their knees. Look for taut bands and painful areas just along and below the iliac crest. Place the leg into extension and adduction off the edge of the table, behind the patient, as shown in figure 12.56. In this position, the anterior gluteus medius can be treated without having to compress through the gluteus maximus. First, use your elbow to treat the anterior portion of the gluteus medius, pressing in and up toward the iliac crest. When you find a taut band, press on it slowly for two or three breaths, then release.

Next, treat the posterior gluteus medius. Flex and adduct the upper thigh with the leg off the table in front of the patient, as shown in figure 12.57. Press straight into the gluteus medius and up toward the iliac crest and sacrum, giving particular attention to painful and tender areas.

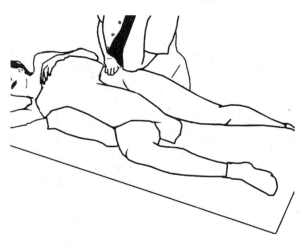

Figure 12.56

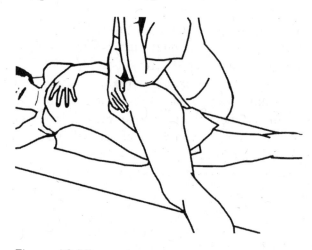

Figure 12.57

Follow compression with contraction and relaxation. Have the patient return their leg to the neutral, straight-leg position while still lying on their side. Use your right hand to resist as the patient presses the upper leg toward the ceiling with 30 percent of their strength, as shown in figure 12.58. Hold this for 15 to 20 seconds, then have the patient exhale and relax. Next, place your hand under the knee and have the patient press down with 30 percent of their strength for 15 to 20 seconds, then have the patient exhale and relax.

Treating the gluteus minimus in the side-lying position: After treating the gluteus medius, where you compressed up toward the iliac crest, have the patient lie in the position shown in figure 12.56, but now treat the gluteus minimus by angling down toward the greater trochanter. You'll be compressing roughly halfway between the iliac crest and the greater trochanter. Angle your elbow toward the greater trochanter from anterior to posterior, treating any painful spots you find. Follow compression with an even more acute stretch by allowing the patient's relaxed upper leg to fall farther off the table.

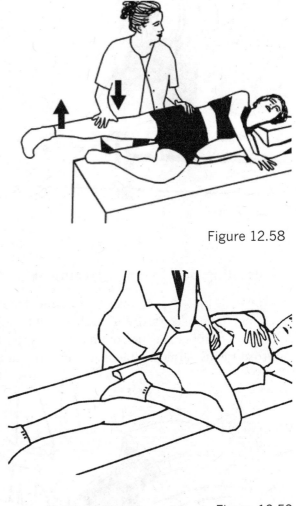

Figure 12.58

Figure 12.59

Treating the piriformis and gluteus maximus in a stretched side-lying position: Have the patient lie on their side with the buttock to be treated on top, as shown in figure 12.59. The lower leg can be left straight. The upper leg is bent with both hip and knee in flexion, and adducted so the knee is resting on the treatment table. If the patient isn't able to achieve this stretched position, place pillows under the upper leg to decrease adduction until they feel comfortable. Unlike normal muscle fibers, taut bands won't stretch, so you can find them more easily with the patient in this stretched position. To treat the gluteus maximus and the piriformis, start by palpating the stretched gluteus maximus, looking for taut bands along the posterior two-thirds of the iliac crest and along the sacrum and coccyx. Work forward to the anterior attachment on the tensor fasciae latae, feeling for any taut bands and applying compression wherever you find them.

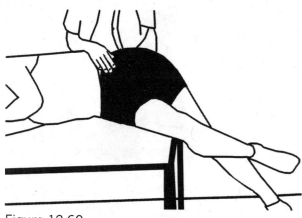

Figure 12.60

Advanced treatment in the side-lying position: Have the patient lie on their side with both legs hanging off the end of the treatment table, as shown in figure 12.60. This is an extremely effective position for treating the gluteus medius and gluteus minimus, as well as the tensor fasciae latae. Because of the degree of stretch inherent in the position, use less compressive force and remain in constant communication with the patient so you don't keep them in this position any longer than is tolerable.

Standing Bent over the Treatment Table

Have the patient bend over the treatment table in a relaxed position. An adjustable treatment table (preferably with electrically controlled height adjustment) is ideal for this purpose. Or you can use a folded body support cushion or pillows to support the upper body. With the patient in this position, you can treat the uppermost gluteus medius and gluteus maximus. And if you have the patient internally

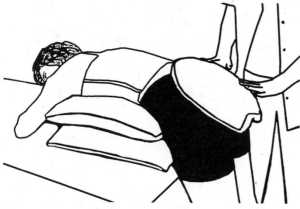

Figure 12.61

and externally rotate the leg, you can evaluate and treat the gluteus medius, gluteus minimus, and piriformis while they're shortened or stretched. This position also allows isolation of hip extension so you can evaluate contractile effort of the gluteus maximus and hamstrings with minimal stress to the lumbar vertebrae. (This is the preferred position if prone hip extension is too painful for the patient's lumbar vertebrae or sacrum.) If compression is too painful in this bent-over position, try treating the buttocks through a heated Mother Earth Pillow, as shown in figure 12.61.

Treatment with Active Contraction

Compression of a muscle after it's been actively shortened is a good way to retrain the muscle and facilitate its full function. The most effective time to bring about changes and normalize the muscle is during focused relaxation after contraction. We often alternate compression treatment with contraction or active use of the muscles.

On Hands and Knees

With the patient on their hands and knees, you can isolate the piriformis, the anterior fibers of the gluteus medius and gluteus minimus, and the gogos. After treating the patient in a side-lying position, have them get on their hands and knees on the treatment table. Have them lift the leg being treated out to the side while keeping the knee bent, as shown in figure 12.62. Repeat this three to five times, then return to a side-lying position. Assess the muscles again. You should find the tissue softer.

On Hands and Knees with Resistance

With the patient on their hands and knees, apply gentle resistance to the outside of the thigh, as shown in figure 12.62, as the patient raises the leg being treated outward using 30 percent of their strength. Hold for 10 to 20 seconds, then have the patient exhale and relax. After repeating this three times, the patient should lie on their side while you assess and treat the gluteus medius, gluteus minimus, and piriformis.

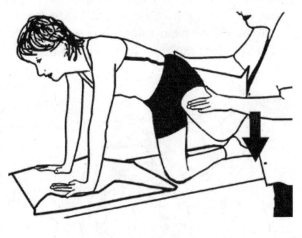

Figure 12.62

Active Contraction of Opposer Muscles During Treatment

We've found it beneficial to treat the buttock muscles while alternately contracting the hip flexors (iliopsoas and rectus femoris) and extensors (the hamstrings and gluteal muscles). Because muscles with chronic trigger points are tight and lack local circulation, you can help reverse this process by having the patient actively use the muscles during treatment. You can take this a step further by also contracting the opposer muscles, which encourages the primary muscle to relax. Let's look at some examples.

Contracting the Hip Flexors and Extensors

First, assess the flexibility of the gluteal muscles and hamstrings. Bring one knee toward the patient's chest and measure the distance from the upper part of the patella to the chest. While the thigh is still flexed, place one hand on the front of the thigh and the other hand on the back of the thigh. Have the patient press their thigh forward for 5 seconds and then backward for 5 seconds with 30 percent of their strength as you resist the effort. Repeat this at least three times, and after the final sequence, have the patient exhale and relax completely. Press the thigh and knee toward the chest and see if the gluteus maximus is able to stretch any further than before. Note that contraction of the hip flexor muscles can also inhibit full flexion of the thigh, so check the iliopsoas and rectus femoris to make sure they're relaxed. If they aren't, they need to be treated as well.

Active Contraction of Hip Abductors and Adductors

Since there's such an intimate antagonistic relationship between the abductors and adductors, it's imperative that you palpate and assess the status of both. With the patient supine, flex one leg at the hip and knee while the other leg remains straight on the table. Allow the bent leg to fall open, and palpate the outer portion of the gluteal muscles to see if they're contracting in this passive, shortened position. Next, bring the leg into adduction and palpate to see if the adductors are contracting in this passive, shortened position. If there is restriction or pain while the leg is being either passively abducted or passively adducted, this means the adductors or abductors need to be treated.

To use active contraction, relaxation, and stretching for these muscles, place one hand on the inside of the knee and the other hand on the outside of the knee and ask the patient to use 30 percent of their strength to abduct, then adduct, the thigh as you resist, contracting for 10 seconds in each direction. Repeat this sequence three times, then retest to determine if the same muscles are no longer contracting when passively shortened, and if they can stretch further without pain.

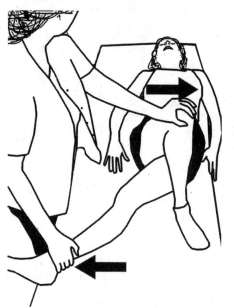

Figure 12.63

Supine Gluteus Medius and Gluteus Minimus Stretch

With patient supine, bend the right knee and hip and place the patient's right foot on the left side of the left thigh, as shown in figure 12.63. While standing to the right of the patient, pull the left leg toward you until you feel some resistance. Next, ask the patient to pull the leg against your hand using 30 percent of their strength for 15 seconds, and then have them push the leg against your hand for another 15 seconds. Ask the patient to relax for a few seconds, then have them repeat the contractions in both directions two more times, holding for 10 seconds and then for 5 seconds, and relaxing after each set.

Combined Spray and Stretch

The spray patterns for the various buttock muscles are very similar, but the positioning of the patient can vary depending on which muscle you're focusing on. The position of the patient should optimally stretch the muscle you wish to focus on and allow for full lengthening after the stretching, relaxing, and reheating have occurred.

The muscles should be taken to the greatest pain-free stretch achievable using the positions shown in the figures below. Spray the vapocoolant over the area following the patterns outlined in the illustrations. The spray pattern for all these muscles originates at the sacral or ischial border and proceeds outward to varying distances down the hip and thigh and, for some, onto the lower leg. Slow, steady sweeps should be applied as the patient simultaneously exhales and further relaxes. At the same time, gently increase the stretch, but not to the point of pain. After spraying the vapocoolant, immediately apply heat over the area, using warm Fomentek bags, Mother Earth Pillows, or hydrocollator packs. This heating further relaxes the patient and facilitates their ability to stretch. Then have the patient move the muscle through its full range of motion.

Spray and Stretch for the Gluteus Maximus

We'll begin with the most superficial of the gluteal muscles, the gluteus maximus. Note that spray and stretch of this muscle, as shown in figure 12.64, will often restore full pain-free range of motion to all the gluteal muscles, even those much deeper in the buttocks. The stretched position for treatment of the gluteus maximus also stretches the posterior segment of the gluteus medius and gluteus minimus, as well as the piriformis. If you've determined through testing that those muscles harbor trigger points, you should continue down the leg to cover the full pain referral pattern (see figures 12.65 through 12.67 for the other spray patterns).

With the patient relaxed and fully supported, replicate the position shown in figure 12.64, with the patient lying on their side with the top leg flexed at the hip and knee as much as possible without pain, and the knee resting on the treatment table. Spray the entire buttock and down the leg and ask the patient to relax completely as you do so. As the muscles relax, gently press the knee closer to the chest to further flex the hip. Then apply heat and have the patient perform a few cycles of active range of motion, bringing the hip into fully shortened and lengthened positions. This can be done as the patient lies on their side or while standing.

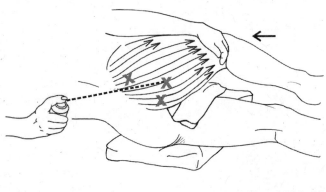

Figure 12.64

Including the Paraspinals in Spray and Stretch

Since the paraspinals can harbor trigger points that refer pain into the gluteal muscles, which in turn can cause satellite activation in the gluteal muscles, it makes sense to spray the paraspinal and gluteal muscles while the patient is in a seated position or standing bent over.

For the seated position, a stool is best. The patient should be seated and hunched all the way over, with their fingers touching the floor between their legs (see figure 6.36 in chapter 6, Paraspinals). Before spraying, have the patient inhale and look upward, then have them exhale and bend forward fully as you apply the cold spray. Apply the spray in sweeps starting at the mid-thoracic back and continuing downward onto the buttocks. Immediately afterward, apply heat to help the patient achieve a greater relaxed stretch.

Another version of this position has the patient in the long sitting position on the treatment table (see figure 6.34 in chapter 6, Paraspinals). This will further stretch the hamstrings and gluteus maximus. Spray from the mid-thoracic back downward over the buttocks. For both positions, the spray should be applied on both sides of the spine. Immediately afterward, apply heat and then encourage an increased stretch with a careful, gentle press on the back.

Spray and Stretch for the Gluteus Medius and Gluteus Minimus

To treat the gluteus medius and gluteus minimus, have the patient lying on their side with varying degrees of straight-leg hip extension and flexion accompanied by internal or external rotation and

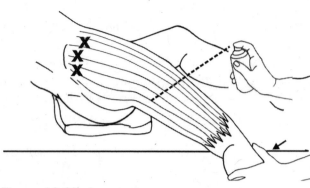

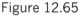

Figure 12.65

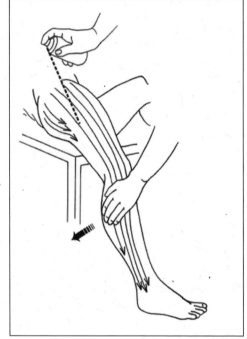

Figure 12.66

adduction. The spray pattern is essentially the same for the gluteus medius and gluteus minimus, except that for the gluteus minimus, if the patient has the complete referral pattern down into the lateral lower leg and ankle, you should apply the spray over that entire area.

To treat the anterior-most fibers of the gluteus medius, gently encourage the thigh into extension and allow it to hang off the back of the treatment table, as shown in figure 12.65. Treating the gluteus minimus is similar, but in this case the thigh is rotated out and hangs off the end of the treatment table, as shown in figure 12.66. Don't keep the patient in either of these positions very long. After spraying, rewarming, and a further stretch, have the patient stand and take the muscles into full range of motion by turning their toes inward and outward, and then abducting and adducting the thigh.

To treat the posterior-most fibers of the gluteus medius and gluteus minimus, keep the leg straight and flexed about 30 degrees at the hip. Rotate it medially and allow it to hang off the front edge of the treatment table. For the backmost fibers of the gluteus minimus, keep the leg straight, allowing it to drop down a bit and supporting it with one hand as you spray with the other.

Spray and Stretch for the Piriformis

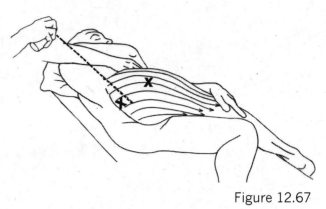

Have the patient lie on their side with as much hip flexion and adduction as possible without pain, as shown in figure 12.67, as this will stretch the piriformis. Get a firm grip on the pelvis and pull back on it while the patient uses their own hand to press down on the outside of the knee. As the patient exhales and relaxes, apply sweeps of the cold spray from the sacral border, over the buttocks, and onto the thigh. When maximum stretch is achieved, apply heat to the area. Next, have the patient move the hip into full adduction and abduction while it's flexed, and to full internal and external rotation while it's straight, repeating the entire series at least three times.

Figure 12.67

Summary

After treatment and retesting the patient for range of motion, ask the patient to describe their post-treatment pain level on a scale of 0 to 10. If treatment is done properly, the patient should experience a significant increase in range of motion and reduction in pain after no more than two or three treatments.

Chapter 13

Hamstrings

Hamstrings is the term commonly used to refer to a group of three muscles in the back of the thigh: the *semitendinosus*, the *semimembranosus*, and the *biceps femoris*. Trigger points in the hamstrings refer pain to the lower buttocks and contribute to low back pain by restricting normal movement of the pelvis. Muscles need movement to stay pain free and maintain full function. When trigger points in the hamstrings limit the range of motion of the pelvis, this has a cascade effect, limiting movement in the low back, waist, abdomen, and hips. The end result is often chronic pain in the upper and lower back, hips, thighs, legs, and even the neck and shoulders.

Drs. Travell and Simons nicknamed the hamstrings and related muscles "chair-seat victims" for a simple reason: When you're seated, especially if your legs don't rest easily on the floor or a footrest, the front of the chair seat pushes into your hamstrings. This is particularly a problem for shorter people, for whom normal chairs are often too large. The front edge of the chair can compress the hamstrings to the point of reducing blood flow and even causing nerve compression. When prolonged, this activates trigger points in the backs of the thighs. All too often, the result is reduced mobility of the pelvis and other muscles in both the front and back of the torso.

A healthy pelvis moves in all directions. If the muscles in the front of the thighs are chronically shortened and tight, they can tip the pelvis forward. In contrast, if the hamstrings, running down the backs of the thighs, are chronically tight, this can tilt the pelvis backward. When the pelvis is tipped either backward or forward continuously, it causes stresses in the torso and neck that can flatten the low back, causing the head to lean forward and also activating trigger points in some of the torso and hip muscles. The ultimate consequence of this long chain of causation is back and buttocks pain.

Where Are the Hamstrings and What Do They Do?

The semitendinosus and semimembranosus make up the inside of the back of the thigh, as shown in figure 13.1. The biceps femoris has two heads, one long and one short. The long head of the biceps femoris makes up the outside of the back of the thigh; and though it may seem strange, the short head isn't considered part of the hamstrings. All three hamstring muscles start at the bones we sit on—the ischial tuberosities—and run down the backs of the thighs to just below the knee on either side of the lower leg bones, the tibia on the inside and the fibula on the outside.

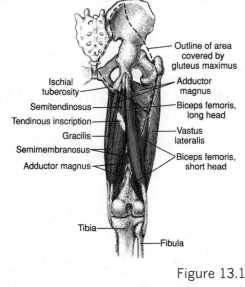

The hamstrings are three of the longer muscles in the body, crossing over both the hip and the knee. When contracted, the hamstrings move the thigh backward and extend the hips, and also flex the knee to bring the heel toward the buttocks. They also help hold the bottom of the pelvis down. In addition, the semitendinosus and semimembranosus rotate the leg inward, and the biceps femoris rotates the thigh outward. The hamstrings also help support us in an upright position when we stand, walk, or run. And finally, they help stabilize movement when we bend forward while standing.

Figure 13.1

Hamstring Pain Referral Patterns

Most commonly, trigger points in the hamstrings refer pain upward to the bottom of the buttock, as shown in figure 13.2. Less often, the same trigger points can refer pain to the back of the thigh, knee, and calf. Because of this pattern, referred pain from trigger points in the hamstring muscles can easily be mistaken for true sciatica.

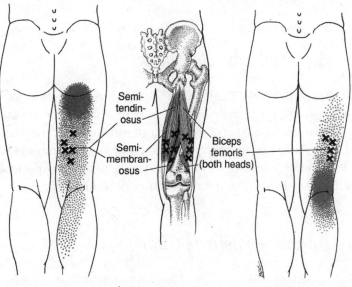

In addition to tipping the pelvis backward, chronically short hamstrings also cause pain at the junction of the muscle and tendon or pain where the tendon attaches to the bone (tendonitis). Chronically tight hamstrings place greater stress on these attachments. When this happens, first there is tenderness in the area of the attachment, which can develop trigger points (known as attachment trigger points). When tightness persists, it may cause bone spurs or calcification. This can sometimes become sufficiently developed to be detectible in X-rays or MRIs.

Figure 13.2

Effective trigger point treatment and restoration of normal range of motion usually eliminates the pressure on the tendinous attachments. Not only does this help with the pain or swelling, it can actually cause the bone spur to recede to the point where it isn't visible on X-rays. If this seems strange, remember that bones are living tissue, not merely a static framework for the living body; they interact with the muscles and respond to trauma, constant pulling from chronically shortened muscles, and changes in the health of the muscles. Bone spurs are an abnormal phenomenon, caused by abnormal stress on the musculoskeletal system. Elimination of that stress will usually get rid of the pain of tendonitis and, in some cases, the calcification itself.

What Aggravates the Hamstrings?

By far the most common activity leading to hamstring problems is too much sitting. No matter how well adapted your seating is, you need to move around regularly to avoid chronically tightened hamstrings.

Pressure from the Front of the Chair Seat

Suppose you avoid prolonged sitting. You still need to consider the chairs you sit in. When the front edge of a chair presses into the middle to lower part of the hamstrings, it can activate trigger points, which in turn may cause a deep aching pain in the buttocks, the thighs, or the backs of the knees and calves. The chair edge can also compress peripheral nerves in the thighs, causing tingling and numbness. Fortunately, this nerve compression is generally mild and the symptoms usually go away once you stop using the chair that causes it. However, the trigger points may persist.

If you can't easily slide your hand between the chair seat and your thighs, the chair doesn't fit you properly. Switch to an adjustable chair that permits you to change the height of the seat or to angle the seat bottom downward toward the front, or get an angled footrest that will elevate your hamstrings off the seat.

Adaptive Muscle Change

Too much sitting can cause the leg muscles to develop what we call "adaptive trigger points." In other words, the hamstrings say to themselves, "Fine, if you want to sit so much, I'll just shorten myself a little to make it easier." So if you sit most of the time, these muscles may adapt themselves to a constantly shortened length. If you then try to use the muscle fully lengthened, in the way it was intended, for walking, running, or jumping, you're likely to experience the unhappy results: hamstring "pulls," referred pain, or very restricted range of motion.

Adaptive Postural Change

Another problem with sitting so much is that it keeps the knees bent most of the time. Many of us retain this bent position to a small degree when we stand up. Then, to compensate for the bent knees, the torso bends forward to maintain balance. This can cause stress on the superficial paraspinal muscles, quadratus lumborum, iliopsoas, and abdominals, as well as other muscles not covered in this book. As a result, these muscles can all develop active trigger points, which then refer pain to the lower back and buttocks. This can develop even further to activation of trigger points in the gluteal muscles, including the piriformis, which can lead to compression of the sciatic nerve.

This chain of causation may seem bewilderingly complex. Suffice it to say that too much sitting or an incorrect seated posture can affect the entire pelvic region and torso. So don't ignore your hamstrings—even if they don't hurt.

Bed Rest

Bed rest may be a good remedy for some conditions, but it can cause problems for the hamstrings. The normal movements involved in standing, walking, and running help keep the hamstrings in good condition. Prolonged bed rest is one of the worst things, not only for the hamstrings, but also for other muscles that refer pain to the low back. If you must have prolonged bed rest for other reasons, you should engage in movement therapy if at all possible.

Structural Imbalances

Many people have a pelvic structure that's smaller on one side than the other, known as a small hemipelvis. The difference might be as little as 1/8 inch or more than 3/4 inch. It usually goes undiagnosed because very few physicians look for it. If you have this condition, you're probably unaware of it, but it will manifest itself in various ways. For example, to maintain yourself in a balanced upright position when sitting, you may tend to lean forward so most of your weight is on your thighs (hamstrings) instead of your sit bones. Another common method of adjusting for this is to sit with your legs crossed, thereby lifting the smaller side up. This causes most of your weight to be supported by the opposite thigh, which often activates trigger points in the hamstrings on the weight-bearing side. (See Mechanical Factors, in chapter 17, for details.)

Acute Overload

When you lift objects while keeping your knees straight, you can develop trigger points in the hamstrings (and the soleus). These trigger points can refer pain to the sacrum and the buttocks and can also mimic the pain pattern of sciatica.

Car Accidents

Regardless of the direction of impact, car accidents sometimes activate hamstring trigger points, especially in the area referring pain to the buttocks.

Excessive Strengthening Exercise

Some fitness enthusiasts like to do exercises focused on strengthening the hamstring muscles. Doing this to excess without adequate stretching can shorten the hamstrings and make them very sore. And when you resume a seated position after exercise, the muscles will adapt to this shortened position and become unable to lengthen normally when you walk or run. Riding a bike with the seat too low can have the same result.

Do I Have Trigger Points in My Hamstrings?

Chronically shortened hamstrings are so prevalent in the general population that testing is almost unnecessary. You probably have trigger points in the hamstrings if you have pain in the back of your thighs, and you definitely have trigger points if pressing on specific painful spots refers pain to the buttock, the back or side of the thigh, or the back of the knee or calf. (See figure 13.2, above, for the most likely spots to find these hamstring trigger points.) Also, if your hamstrings are chronically shortened, which is very common among adults, you're likely to have trigger points in the hamstrings. For a simple test that can help you answer the question of whether you have trigger points in your hamstrings, see the standing toe touch test in chapter 6 (page 78). In addition, the following fairly common conditions are all positive indicators for trigger points in the hamstrings.

Snapping bottom syndrome. When the hamstring is chronically contracted, its attachment tendon may flip back and forth over the sit bones, which is quite painful. This is sometimes called *snapping bottom syndrome*; it may also be referred to as *hamstring tendonitis* or *tenosynovitis*. If you've been given any of these diagnoses, proper treatment of tight hamstrings is likely to alleviate your condition.

Problems after surgery. After nerve root decompression surgery, it's very common to find active trigger points in the hamstrings and other muscles. Often the surgery is a success from the point of view of the surgeon but a failure in the final analysis because the patient still has pain. And sometimes the pain and dysfunction are worse after surgery than before. "Failure" is a fair word to describe many back surgeries. In fact, it's so common that it has a name in the medical lexicon: failed back surgery syndrome. You can find articles advising surgeons on how to deal with this when it occurs. If the myofascial component (which doesn't show up on X-rays or MRIs) were also addressed, the overall success rate might be significantly improved. Some types of back surgery are regarded, even within the profession, as basically a crapshoot. Since conventional doctors generally don't consider myofascial trigger points as a possible cause of chronic back pain, you'll need to consider it on your own, either before or after surgery.

Sciatica. If you've been diagnosed with sciatica, you probably have active hamstring trigger points. Effective treatment of these trigger points may partially or completely alleviate the sciatic pain.

Collapsing leg syndrome. Perhaps you have collapsing leg syndrome, a scary condition in which the leg seems to give out without warning. This is usually due to trigger points in the thigh muscles that cause them to suddenly contract, which in turn can cause the knee to flex or collapse. Again, trigger point treatment can generally alleviate this condition completely and fairly quickly (Travell and Simons 1992).

Other Symptoms Pointing to Hamstring Trigger Points

Other common problems include limping and pain in the buttocks when walking and even when sitting. You may feel buttocks pain when getting out of a chair or after uncrossing your legs. Another common problem is buttocks pain when trying to sleep.

With chronically contracted hamstrings, there's a tendency to fall forward when walking rapidly. Running, walking on uneven surfaces, hopping, dancing, and jumping are all difficult or impossible. Those with chronically contracted hamstrings generally avoid these activities, and also avoid bending forward for fear of falling. Unfortunately, this fear of movement further restricts mobility of the pelvis, which exacerbates back and buttocks pain and can eventually result in semiparalysis. Remember, movement is the key to healthy muscles.

A less frequent consequence of compressed hamstrings is a condition known as thrombophlebitis, or impaired blood flow. In most cases, this constriction of blood flow is limited to the superficial veins. However, if it continues, it can lead to more serious impairment and even an embolism. While there are several possible causes of this condition, one is chronic excessive pressure on the hamstrings due to an ill-fitting chair or poor seated posture.

Children of all ages can have trigger points, too. "Growing pains" in small children are actually often due to trigger points in the hamstrings. Even infants can be afflicted, as they're often seated with their legs dangling or unsupported. This can lead to trigger points that cause restlessness, squirming, and crying.

Helpful Hints for Eliminating Trigger Points in the Hamstrings

Beyond self-care, attention to a few simple ergonomic issues can go a long way toward alleviating trigger points in the hamstrings:

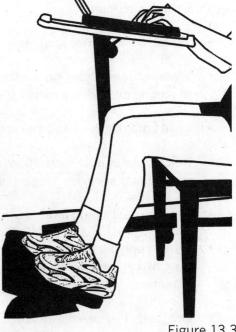

- **Don't overbend your knees.** You may have to sit for much of the day, but don't make it worse by bending your knees at an acute angle. Placing your feet under your chair puts the hamstrings in an extreme shortened position. A footrest can raise your thighs off the edge of the chair seat. For best results, use an angled footrest, as shown in figure 13.3. This extends the legs a bit and gently stretches the backs of the lower legs.

- **Use a standing desk.** If you have chronically tight muscles in your neck, back, abdomen, hips, or legs, particularly the hamstrings, buy a standing desk, which will allow you to work in a standing position. Another alternative is a desk that can be adjusted to

Figure 13.3

different heights, so you can alternate between standing and sitting. When standing at a desk, it helps to raise one leg, as shown in figure 13.4, or to stretch one leg backward, as shown in figure 13.5. Use these positions for each leg, and keep varying your position in order to stretch the shortened hamstring muscles.

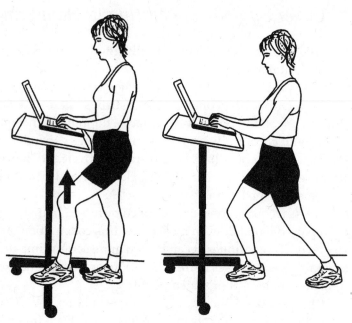

- **Make sure your furniture fits you.** A majority of the population has chronically shortened hamstrings. If you have persistent low back and buttock pain and dysfunction, you should consider every chair you use during the day—at work or at home. It could make a significant difference and help you eliminate the pain.

Figure 13.4   Figure 13.5

Self-Care Treatment

Here are a few general pointers to keep in mind for all the compression techniques and stretches described in this chapter:

- Warm the area prior to treatment, especially when your symptoms are severe.

- When sitting or lying on the floor for any form of self-care (compression, stretching, range of motion exercises), a carpeted surface is ideal; alternatively, you can use an exercise mat.

- Treat both thighs even if you appear to have trigger points on only one side.

- Refer to the muscle illustrations and compress all areas indicated by X's. The larger X's represent likely spots for trigger points, but the entire muscle requires treatment.

- Never exceed a pain level of 6 on a scale of 0 to 10.

- When applying compression, sustain the compression for up to 30 seconds and repeat at least two or three times, or until there's a noticeable decrease in pain and increase in range of motion.

- Gradually increase the amount of compression as you feel the muscle softening and relaxing. Be aware of how the tissues respond to treatment.

- When stretching, hold the position for two to three normal breaths.

- When a stretch is repeated several times on both sides, alternate sides with each repetition.

- After treatment and stretching, do the range of motion exercises for the hamstrings in chapter 16.

Compression

Take a good look at figure 13.6. The large X's mark the spots most likely to have trigger points. However, we recommend you compress the entire area, because tight, painful spots can be found anywhere in the hamstrings.

It's a good idea to warm the area prior to compression. Try using warm Mother Earth Pillows or Fomentek bags on the backs of the thighs, as shown in figure 13.7, for 10 minutes before beginning compression. You can use different tools and techniques to look for these trigger points, which are distributed among the semimembranosus, semitendinosus, and biceps femoris. Start by using your fingers to slowly press into all the areas marked with small X's to evaluate and treat them simultaneously. Palpate the entire muscle, looking for taut bands and painful spots.

Next, stand up and feel the attachment on your ischial tuberosity, or sit bone. Then take a look at figure 13.1, above, to see where the semitendinosus and semimembranosus attach to the larger lower leg bone (the tibia) and where the biceps femoris attaches to the smaller lower leg bone (the fibula). As you sit down again, feel the places where they attach to the lower leg, looking for tender, painful, tight spots.

You can use a variety of tools, including a Jacknobber, Backnobber, foam roller, tennis ball, hard rubber ball, baseball, softball, or compression therapy ball. The choice of tool depends on your strength, your pain tolerance, and what's available. Larger balls, with a 5- to 7-inch diameter, work better at the beginning, when you may be very tender and need gentle pressure. As your pain level decreases, try tools that provide more spot-specific pressure, such as the Jacknobber and Backnobber, and smaller, harder balls.

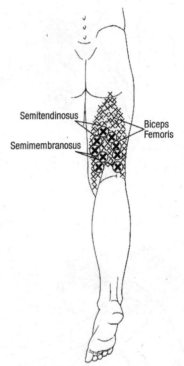

MYO compression for Hamstrings

Figure 13.6

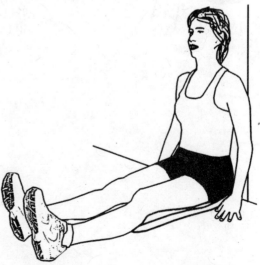

Figure 13.7

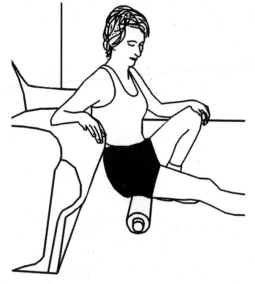

Figure 13.8

Beginner Level

A great tool to use on the back of the thighs is a foam roller with a 4-inch diameter. Start with your torso supported on a couch or a sturdy chair, with the leg you're treating extended and the other leg bent, as shown in figure 13.8. Place the roller under the sit bone on the side with the extended leg and move the roller toward the back of the knee, feeling for taut bands and painful spots. Wherever you find a painful spot, stop moving and relax into the roller for 10 to 30 seconds. Proceed in this way along the full length of the back of the thigh. Because compression from the roller is fairly diffused, it should be tolerable and very beneficial to treat the hamstrings in this way. However, if the compression is too painful at first, you can use a warm Fomentek bag over the roller or place one or more thick towels over the roller to make it softer.

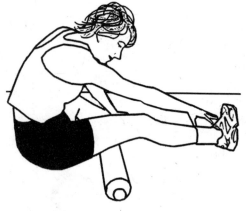

Figure 13.9

Intermediate Level

Adding a stretch will intensify the previous treatment. It's also easier to locate taut bands when you stretch while doing compression. First, sit on the floor with the leg you're treating extended and the other leg bent, and compress your hamstring with a 4-inch foam roller, as described above. Then, flex your torso forward at the waist, reaching toward the toes of your extended leg and using your other hand to maintain your balance, as shown in figure 13.9. Again, wherever you find painful spots, stop and relax into the roller for 10 to 30 seconds.

Advanced Level

After you've done self-care for two to three weeks, your pain level should be noticeably lower. At that point, try using a Jacknobber. A good position for doing this is seated with your back against a wall. Start by rolling sideways to place most of your weight onto your opposite hip, and place the Jacknobber under the back of your thigh as high as you can, up near your sit bone, as shown in figure 13.10. Gently lean your body weight into the Jacknobber, feeling for taut, painful spots and moving the Jacknobber from spot to spot by hand. Wherever you find a tender spot, allow your leg to relax down onto the tool slowly until you feel moderate discomfort, then hold that position for 10 to 30 seconds. As the pain abates, press a little harder onto the tool, remembering to breathe and relax as you continue the compression. Repeat this compression down the leg until you've treated all the painful areas on the back of the thigh.

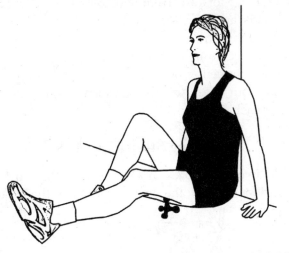

Figure 13.10

Stretching

No matter how tight your hamstrings are, you can always start with a gentle stretch and then gradually intensify it as you begin to restore mobility to the muscle. The hamstrings are big muscles. For many of us, they are so tight and immobile due to too much sitting that they're almost in a shut-down state. Stretching is extremely important to counteract this, so we offer many options below. If you vary your stretches you'll have more fun, and you'll recover faster too. Keep in mind that it helps to warm the hamstrings before stretching. All of the stretches described below are suitable for beginners.

Seated Flat-Back Hamstring Stretch

This stretch is easier to do at first with one leg bent and the other straight. So start with the left leg bent and the right leg straight. Sit on the floor with your back against a wall for support. Start with a warm Mother Earth Pillow or Fomentek bag under your right thigh. Press your back and head against the wall. Notice how straight your back is, and try to maintain this flat-backed position as you flex your entire torso forward, bending only at the hips. If you round your back, you'll be stretching your back muscles, not your hamstrings. If you do this correctly, you'll feel the stretch in your hamstring all the way from your sit bone to your knee. Remember to breathe slowly, and each time you exhale, try to bring your torso a little closer to your thigh. Do this stretch slowly at least three times for each leg, keeping your back flat.

To add the contraction and relaxation components, bend your right knee slightly and press your right heel into the floor with 30 percent of your strength. Hold the contraction for about 15 seconds. Relax as you exhale slowly, then straighten your leg, reach toward your toes (again, keeping your back flat), and try to stretch a little farther. Do this on both sides.

Seated Flat-Back Stretch with Legs Apart

This variation on the previous stretch focuses on areas that refer pain to the buttocks. While sitting on the floor with your back flat against the wall as before, spread your legs apart at a 60-degree angle, then bend forward from your hips toward your left foot as far as you comfortably can. Hold for 10 seconds, and then slowly return to the starting position.

Do this stretch three times toward each foot, alternating sides and striving for a slightly greater stretch each time without pushing beyond a level of moderate discomfort. Finally, do the same stretch toward the center, between your legs, three times. Remember to keep your back straight and bend only from your hips. Add the contraction and relaxation components described in the previous exercise after each stretch.

Hamstring Stretch in a Doorway

Lie on your back in a doorway with your left leg up against the wall and your right leg flat on the floor through the doorway (or keep the knee bent if that's more comfortable). Place your left foot

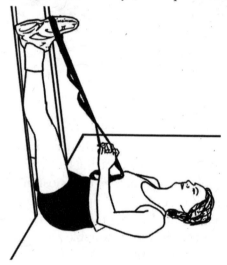

through the loop of a stretching strap and hold the other end in your hand, as shown in figure 13.11. If your hamstrings are very tight, this position may put your hamstring in more of a stretch than you can stand, even as a starting point. If so, move away from the wall, as shown in figure 13.12.

Next, try to pull your left leg toward your head with the strap while keeping your knee straight, as shown in figure 13.13. Breathe and relax as you do this. Each time you exhale, try to bring your leg a little closer to your head, and keep trying for a little more stretch until you feel as much strain as you can comfortably stand. Do this stretch at least three times for each leg, letting your leg rest against the wall for at least 10 seconds after each stretch.

Figure 13.11

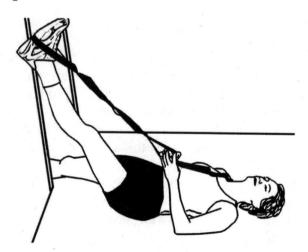

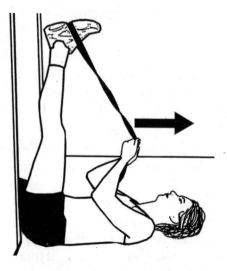

Figure 13.12   Figure 13.13

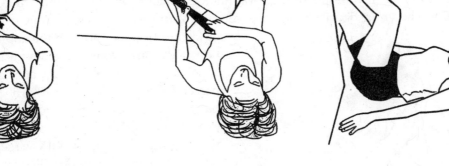

Figure 13.14   Figure 13.15   Figure 13.16

For variation, drop your leg to the side and pull toward a point outside your shoulder, as shown in figure 13.14. Do this stretch three times for each leg, each time dropping the leg slightly farther to the side as shown in figure 13.15. Intersperse your stretches with gentle contractions, bending your leg slightly at the knee, as shown in figure 13.16, and pressing your heel into the wall with 30 percent of your strength. Hold the contraction for 15 seconds, then exhale slowly and resume the stretch, trying to pull your leg a little farther away from the wall than previously.

Seated Hamstring Stretch

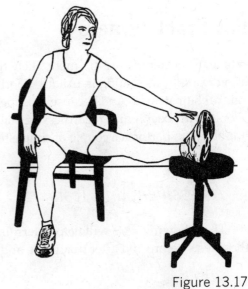

Sit on a comfortable chair with your right foot on the floor and your left leg out to the side supported by another chair or footstool, as shown in figure 13.17. While keeping your back flat, lean your entire torso toward your left foot, bending at the hip. Breathe slowly, and as you exhale, try to stretch a little farther, remembering to keep your back straight. Repeat this three times for each leg, each time reaching a bit farther toward your foot as you exhale. You may not be able to stretch very far at all to start. Don't worry; just try to reach toward your foot as much as your tight hamstrings will permit with only mild discomfort. Doing this exercise daily, together with other self-care treatments, will increase your flexibility over time.

Figure 13.17

For a variation, start from the same position and flex forward between your legs instead of toward the foot of the extended leg. This stretches the inner portion of the hamstrings. Repeat three times.

Contract and Relax with a Partner

A good way to contract and relax the hamstrings is with help from a partner, if available. Lie on your back on the floor or a bed and have your partner lift your right leg up, keeping it straight, until you feel some resistance in your hamstrings. Maintain that height and place your ankle on your partner's shoulder as shown in figure 13.18. Depending on your partner's height, they can stand closer or farther from you to give the appropriate elevation. Then push your ankle downward onto their shoulder, contracting your hamstrings with 30 percent of your strength for 20 to 30 seconds. Your partner should remain stationary. Relax as you exhale, and remain relaxed as your partner raises your leg slightly higher until you feel resistance in your hamstrings again. You'll usually be able to have it lifted a little higher each time, as muscles generally become a little longer after contraction. In this new, slightly higher resting position, have your partner hold steady as you once again push your ankle downward with 30 percent of your strength. Repeat this contract and relax exercise at least twice for each leg, even if you have painful, tight hamstrings on only one side.

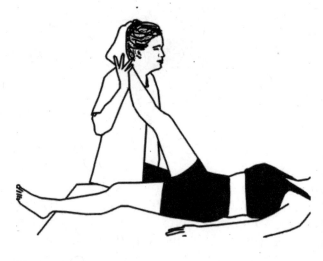

Figure 13.18

For Practitioners

People of shorter stature are more likely than the rest of the population to have tight hamstrings with trigger points, as seating is usually poorly adapted for them, resulting in chronically shortened and painful hamstrings. And because most people sit for much of their day, it's reasonable to assume most people with back pain, regardless of stature, will have hamstring trigger points. However, it's still important to perform a couple of simple hamstring tests.

Assessment and Tests

The following tests will help determine whether trigger points are present in the hamstrings. Use these tests before and after treatment, and record the results to help you measure progress.

Supine Active Leg Extension

This is a great test for the hamstrings. Start with the patient lying supine on the treatment table with one hip flexed at a 90-degree angle and that same knee flexed so that the lower leg is parallel to the table. Have the patient hold the thigh with both hands and try to extend the lower leg as close to straight up as they possibly can. Those with perfectly flexible hamstrings will be able to lift their leg straight up. If they can lift their leg to within about 10 degrees of straight, they probably don't have hamstring restriction. You can use a goniometer (see chapter 3) to measure the angle exactly. If you don't have one, judge and record the angle by eye. Perform this test for both lower limbs.

Single-Thigh Leg Lift

We use this test for hamstring dysfunction, but it is often used to test for vertebral disk dysfunction as well. Have the patient lie supine on the treatment table with a rolled-up towel beneath the lumbar region of their lower back. With the patient as relaxed as possible, slowly lift one leg as close to vertical as possible. Ask the patient to note any painful or tight areas. If they have pain in the lumbar region, this could indicate disk dysfunction. If the pain increases when the patient dorsiflexes the ankle, you may want to refer for orthopedic evaluation.

If there is no restriction or pain and the leg can be raised to close to a 90-degree angle, the hamstrings don't have trigger points. If the patient experiences pain in the hamstrings or the leg can only be raised to an angle of 80 degrees or less, they should be examined for hamstring trigger points. Most people past early adulthood can't pass this test. However, that can also indicate trigger points in the adductor magnus or gastrocnemius (not covered in this book), or the gluteus maximus or paraspinal muscles.

Knee to Armpit Test

The knee to armpit test, described in chapter 5 (page 69), tests for trigger points in the hamstrings, the gluteus maximus, and the iliopsoas.

Standing Toe Touch

This test, described in the first part of this chapter, assesses trigger points and flexibility in the hamstrings, as well as the adductor magnus, gluteus maximus, gastrocnemius, erector spinae, and vastus lateralis. As the patient performs this test, ask them to point out any tight areas. If the patient can touch the floor without pain, there are no active trigger points in the hamstrings or any of the other muscles mentioned above. If they can't reach their toes or if they experience pain in the hamstrings as they attempt to do so, they have active trigger points. Most people past early adulthood cannot pass this test. Do consider the patient's height, weight, and age when deciding whether they pass or fail this test. Use a tape measure to record inches from the tip of the middle finger to the floor. After several treatments, this distance should decrease, indicating increased hamstring flexibility.

Testing Whether the Hamstrings Can Shorten Passively

While most of the tests above help determine the ability of the hamstrings to lengthen properly, it's also important to know whether they can shorten passively without pain, twitching, or cramping, as with a charley horse. To test this, have the patient lie prone on the treatment table. Place one hand on the hamstring you're testing and, with your other hand, passively flex the knee, bringing the heel as close to the buttocks as it will go comfortably. Take care in performing this test, as some patients may experience severe pain when the muscle is shortened beyond a certain point, and the muscle may stay in contraction. Let the patient tell you when you've shortened the muscle enough; once the patient has indicated a pain level of 6 out of 10, don't push the foot farther toward the buttocks. Restriction or pain confirms the need for treatment. Bear in mind that cramping of the hamstring can be very painful. One or two such experiences at your hands can easily persuade a patient to find another health care practitioner.

Sciatic Nerve Complications

Chronically tight hamstrings can lead to an inaccurate diagnosis of sciatica, as pain caused by hamstring trigger points is often felt down the posterior thigh in the distribution of the sciatic nerve, which innervates all three of the hamstring muscles. Since this pattern resembles true sciatic nerve pain, physicians often quite reasonably suspect nerve root compression and order a battery of tests.

Our clinical experience has shown that many cases of this pain pattern, as well as other symptoms, such as numbness and tingling, can be resolved by treating trigger points in the hamstring, gluteal muscles, paraspinals, and quadratus lumborum and correcting underlying perpetuating factors. Since the costs—in time, money, and risk—of myofascial treatment are infinitesimal when compared to surgery, we suggest that myofascial treatment be considered as a first approach, not a last resort, when symptoms of sciatica are present. If myofascial treatment doesn't work, the patient still has the option of surgery.

Treatment Techniques

Treating on the Stretch

One of the best ways to treat the hamstrings is on the stretch, with the patient bent over the treatment table in a relaxed position. An adjustable treatment table (preferably with electrically controlled height adjustment) is ideal for this purpose. Or you can use a folded body support cushion or pillows to support the upper body. The patient's feet should be on the floor with knees straight. The health care practitioner sits on a low stool and treats the hamstrings in this stretched, partially weight-bearing position.

This is a good position to use when a person has hamstring pain or tightening as a result of a sports injury. You can even make this work with a park bench or any stable, raised, flat surface. You can also use this position to finish a treatment as the patient is getting off the table. Whenever you treat the hamstring muscles, try to include some compression on the stretch.

Treating in a Neutral Position

Have the patient lie prone on a body support system, preferably with the hips slightly flexed, with their feet off the end of the treatment table. Don't put bolsters under the ankles, as this shortens the hamstrings. Use your elbow, knuckles, or fingers to apply compression.

Treating in a Shortened Position and While in Range of Motion

Have the patient lie prone on the treatment table on a body support system. With one hand, passively raise the lower leg slowly to a moderate angle (30 to 60 degrees), and compress the hamstring with the other hand or elbow. To treat the muscle through its normal range of motion, simply flex the leg slowly up and down as you apply compression treatment. As you eliminate trigger points, you should note greater range of motion and less sensitivity to treatment.

Stretch, Contract, and Relax

After you've completed compression treatment, always follow with the stretch, contract, and relax sequence. With the patient supine on the treatment table, passively raise one lower limb with extended knee onto your shoulder and gently stretch it for 15 seconds. Ask the patient to contract the hamstring by flexing the knee and pressing the lower leg into your shoulder for 15 seconds, and then relax. Next, stretch the muscle again, raising the leg a little farther toward the ceiling and holding for 10 seconds, then ask the patient to contract the hamstring and press against your shoulder again, this time for 10 seconds. Do this sequence two or three more times, each time reducing the time of contraction slightly. You should notice a definite increase in muscle flexibility when you've completed this stretch, contract, and relax exercise.

Contracting the Antagonist Muscles

Remember that a muscle is more likely to relax after you've contracted the antagonist muscle. In this case, contracting the quads will tend to relax the hamstrings. To do this, have the patient lie prone on the treatment table and ask them to bend their knee as close to 90 degrees as possible, so that the leg points straight up. Place your hand on the anterior ankle and ask the patient to extend the knee, pressing down against your hand for 10 seconds, and then relax.

Another way to contract the quads is to have the patient sit on the edge of the treatment table with their legs dangling down. Place your hand on the anterior ankle and have them extend the knee, pressing the lower leg into your hand for 10 seconds, and then relax.

Another option is to have the patient stretch and contract the quads and the hamstrings alternately using a method known as passive and active rhythmic release. You can do this using the sequence above to contract the quads, and then moving your hand to the posterior ankle and asking the patient to flex the lower leg into your hand. Remember to do all these exercises for both legs, even if the problems occur primarily in one leg.

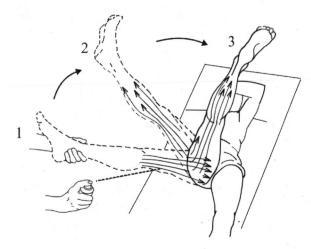

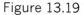

Figure 13.19

Spray and Stretch

Consider using spray and stretch techniques after or alternating with other forms of treatment, particularly if the patient has chronically tight hamstrings and you want to achieve a little more stretching and lengthening of the muscle. You might also use spray and stretch at the end of treatment if there's still some pain and you want to achieve more immediate relief and improved range of motion.

Keep the patient warm, and have a heat source ready to apply to sprayed areas. Start with the patient supine and flexing and adducting the hip with the knee straight, as shown in position 1 in figure 13.19. The thin lines with arrows on the thigh show you where and in what direction to apply the spray. Spray in four parallel lines running distally to proximally, from below the knee toward the groin over the adductors, the semitendinosus, and the semimembranosus toward the pain referral area around the ischial tuberosity. As you spray, flex and abduct at the hip a little farther. Quickly apply heat over the sprayed area for about 30 seconds as you continue to increase hip flexion and abduction.

Then place the patient as shown in position 2 in figure 13.19, with the foot gradually elevated but partly adducting the limb while keeping the hip flexed and knee extended. Note that now the direction of the spray is reversed and goes proximal to distal. Follow the lines and directional arrows. Spray from the accessible gluteal area to the mid-leg in four parallel lines and attempt to increase flexion with each sweep of the spray. Apply heat over the sprayed area while still stretching it and see if you can increase the stretch. Finally, place the patient as shown in position 3 in figure 13.19, with the hip in full flexion and adducted, and spray from the accessible gluteal muscles to the lower leg in four lines over the biceps femoris to the pain referral area on the posterior knee. Immediately after spraying, apply heat while the muscle is still stretched.

Always follow spray and stretch treatment by immediately applying heat to the sprayed areas, and when possible apply heat to the hamstrings for 5 minutes after treatment, with the patient in the seated stretch shown in figure 13.7, above. Conclude treatment with range of motion exercises from the hamstrings protocol in chapter 16. Finally, make sure that patients understand how to do these movements and the importance of making them part of a daily self-care routine.

Chapter 14

Soleus

It may seem strange that a muscle in your lower leg can cause back pain, but in fact, trigger points in certain parts of the soleus can do just that. In the bigger picture, however, soleus trigger points can affect the way you walk, which can be a major perpetuating factor in low back pain. We'll discuss this indirect effect on your walking gait later in this chapter. In our experience, about 15 percent of all cases of chronic low back pain are caused by trigger points in the soleus. And a major perpetuating factor in activation of soleus trigger points is failure to use the lower legs through their full range of motion.

Activation of trigger points in the soleus on the outside of the mid-calf can actually refer pain directly to the low back at the sacroiliac joint, where the sacrum joins the pelvis. But trigger points in other parts of the soleus more often cause heel, foot, or ankle pain. Even so, this pain and tightness in the lower leg and ankle often lead to postural asymmetry or shifts in the way we walk and stand. This can cause severe low back and buttocks pain, which may not necessarily be centered in or near the sacroiliac joint.

This complex interrelationship of pain and dysfunction can make it hard to properly diagnose and treat pain caused by the soleus. We've actually seen a few instances where surgery was performed on the lumbar spinal vertebrae as a means of relieving chronic back pain that was ultimately traced to trigger points and chronic tightness in the soleus muscle. This particular aspect of low back pain is an astonishing example of the complexity and interdependence of the human anatomy. Even chronic headaches, jaw pain, and other facial pain can sometimes ultimately be traced to problems in the lower legs, ankles, and feet. Despite this complexity, it's fairly easy to determine if the soleus is the problem muscle. This chapter offers simple tests to determine if the soleus is a factor in your low back pain.

Where Is the Soleus and What Does It Do?

The soleus is in the back of the lower leg, beneath the gastrocnemius muscle. It starts just below the knee and attaches to the Achilles tendon on the back of the heel bone, as shown in figure 14.1. The soleus

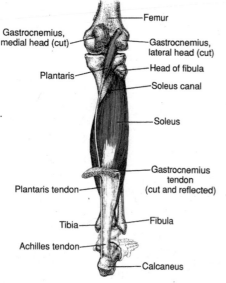

Figure 14.1

helps you push off your toes when walking or jumping. It also helps point your toes and the entire foot downward when cycling, climbing, dancing, walking, or running and assists inversion (turning the sole of the foot inward). Together with the other muscles that point the toes (the plantar flexors), the soleus contributes to ankle and knee stability, especially while walking and running.

The soleus also has an unusual muscular function: It acts as a "second heart." Due to the veins running through it, contracting and relaxing the soleus helps pump blood back to the heart. So it assists in maintaining circulation, something soldiers are thankful for when standing guard duty in the cold. They're actually taught to contract and relax the calf muscles periodically to prevent pooling of blood in the lower legs—and to prevent themselves from passing out and falling over!

Soleus Pain Referral Patterns

The soleus has three trigger point regions, as shown in figure 14.2. The first is about two-thirds of the way down the calf from the back of the knee. Trigger points in this region cause pain in the heel or the Achilles tendon, and sometimes in the bottom of the foot. Trigger points in the second region, located just below the knee, cause pain approximately 3 inches below the knee in the center of the upper calf. Trigger points in the third region, located on the outside of the calf above the ankle, refer pain to the sacroiliac joint on the same side. This third trigger point region is the area that directly refers pain to the lower back.

You need to be aware of the first two referred pain patterns because chronic foot, ankle, and lower leg pain can cause you to modify your gait in ways that affect your posture. This leads to abnormal stress on many of the muscles that directly cause low back pain. So the soleus has both a direct and an indirect influence on low back pain, which, sadly, is lost on most people concerned with treating it.

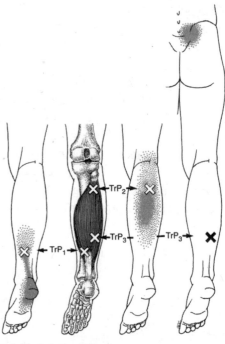

Figure 14.2

What Aggravates the Soleus?

In addition to Morton's foot syndrome (discussed in chapter 17), failure to use the lower legs through their full range of motion frequently activates soleus trigger points. Any of the contributing factors noted below can restrict movement of the lower legs, thereby activating soleus trigger points:

- Wearing high-heeled shoes (especially very high heels)

- Wearing rigid-soled shoes or boots, such as steel-reinforced work boots

- Wearing tight midcalf elastic socks or knee-high stockings

- Wearing slippery socks or smooth-soled slippers on hardwood, tile, or linoleum floors

- Heavy covers on your bed that weigh down your toes and cause the foot to be pointed downward if you sleep on your back

- Standing still for extended periods

- Running or walking on a slanted surface or hiking up a long steep hill

- Frequently bending from the waist with your knees locked straight

- Prolonged driving with your foot pressing on the gas pedal

- Taking long car or plane trips without frequent breaks for walking and stretching

- Resting the calf on an ottoman or footrest with the back of the thigh or knee unsupported

- Sitting on a chair too high to permit your feet to touch the floor, which can restrict blood flow to the soleus

- Excessive ankle pronation due to Morton's foot syndrome or flat feet

Do I Have Trigger Points in My Soleus?

Diminished range of motion in the ankle joint or persistent weakness or pain in the lower legs, heels, feet, or low back are all indications for soleus trigger points. In addition, any of the following problems indicate that trigger points are probably present in the soleus (Travell and Simons 1992):

- Pain and tenderness in the heel

- Inability to put weight on the heel

- Aching in the heel at night

- Painful walking, especially uphill or up and down stairs

- Swelling of the feet and ankles (since trigger points in the soleus can inhibit circulation)

- Inability to squat with heels on the floor

- Limited range of motion in the ankles, making it difficult to pick things up from the floor or lift properly

- Walking like a penguin, with your weight shifting from side to side

- Shortening of your stride when walking

- For children, growing pains in the legs

Tests for Soleus Trigger Points

Can you walk with your knees bent? Can you walk on tiptoe? Can you push off your toes while walking or running? If you answered no to these questions, you probably have soleus trigger points. In addition, here are three simple tests that will help you determine whether you have soleus trigger points: the squat test, the standing toe touch test, and the single heel rise test.

Squat Test

When doing the squat test, you'll need to hold on to a doorjamb or other sturdy support to help maintain stability. Squat down and attempt to touch your buttocks to your calves and upper heels while keeping your feet flat on the floor, as shown in figure 14.3. **Caution:** If this is painful or puts too much strain on your calves and Achilles tendons, stop the test. If you can bring your buttocks down to your heels, you have excellent range of motion. The greater the distance from your buttocks to your heels, the more likely it is that you have trigger points in the soleus muscle.

However, it should be noted that with advancing age, most people lose some range of motion. So the older you are, the more likely it is your buttocks will be some distance from your heels. You should note that tight quadriceps muscles (in the front of the thighs) or problems with your knees could also prevent you from passing this test. As you perform the squat, be aware of any tightness in your quadriceps or restriction in your knees that may interfere with normal range of motion.

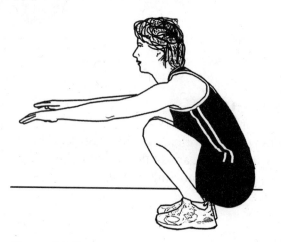

Figure 14.3

Standing Toe Touch Test

For a full description of this test, see chapter 6 (page 78). If you're unable to touch the floor, even with the age allowance, or if you experience pain in your back or legs, you probably have trigger points in your soleus, hamstrings, paraspinal muscles, or gluteus maximus. Keep in mind that tightness or trigger points in any of the muscles of the low back, buttocks, or upper or lower legs can prevent you from touching your toes, so don't rely on this test as the sole basis for determining the presence of trigger points in any specific muscle.

Single Heel Rise Test

This test checks for restriction in the muscles of the back of the calf, including the soleus. While doing this test, you may need to hold on to a sturdy chair or other support. With your shoes off, stand on one foot. With all your weight on that foot, try to rise up onto the ball of the foot. Do one foot at a time. If there's no restriction in the calf muscles, you should be able to rise fully up onto the ball of your foot, as shown in figure 14.4, and maintain that position steadily and without pain for at least 5 seconds. If you're unable to do this, as shown in figure 14.5, that indicates you may have soleus trigger points. In figure 14.5, note how the bottom of the heel is still too close to the floor.

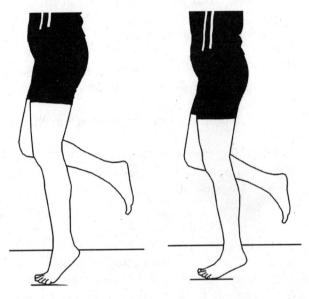

Figure 14.4   Figure 14.5

How Soleus Trigger Points Affect Posture

In normal walking, as you bend and unbend the ankle, the lower leg passes over the center of your foot. If your ankles don't have normal range of motion (the ability to flex and point the foot and to turn in or out), this can shift the placement of your knee or thigh as you walk. This can cause you to shorten your normal stride, preventing the natural swing of the hips. As a result, the muscles that normally move or stabilize these areas can become overused or underused. These changes can affect the way the upper torso sits over the pelvis, which can ultimately affect your neck and head posture. So gradually you don't even notice it, you may begin to walk with shorter strides, bent forward at the waist and with your neck and head stuck out forward. This abnormal gait and posture can cause headaches, jaw pain and dysfunction, or pain in the neck, upper and lower back, buttocks, hips, knees, or feet. It's astonishing to think that problems in the lower legs and feet could cause chronic pain pretty much throughout the body, but we see this quite frequently.

Helpful Hints for Eliminating Trigger Points in the Soleus

Beyond self-care treatments, there are several simple things you can do to alleviate trigger points in the soleus:

- Evaluate for Morton's foot syndrome, and if necessary, purchase proper inserts for the first metatarsal. (See chapter 17 for details.)

- Avoid wearing high heels.

- Get rid of old, worn-out shoes, as they can cause or exacerbate Morton's foot syndrome and activate trigger points in the soleus.

- Avoid tight socks or stockings, which can impair circulation in the lower leg.

- Adjust your bed covers so your feet aren't pressed downward in a pointed position. For example, roll up a large beach towel or blanket and put it near the bottom of your bed, under the covers, alongside your feet to keep most of the weight of the covers off your feet.

- Change your sleeping position as needed to ensure that your legs are in a relaxed, extended, and well-supported position. If you sleep on your side, use a king-size pillow between your legs and keep your legs extended. If you sleep on your back, use a soft pillow under your knees, calves, and feet to improve circulation and help reduce swelling of the feet. (See chapter 17 for details on sleep positions.)

- If your legs feel cold in bed at night, use loose-fitting knee-high or over-the-knee socks to prevent activation of trigger points in the soleus due to chilling.

- If you must stand for long periods (such as at a factory job), vary your stance periodically. Shift your weight from leg to leg, stand on tiptoes or lean back on your heels, stand with your knees slightly bent, or stand with your toes in, and then with your toes out.

- Always walk using your full range of motion, rolling forward through the entire foot, and stop and do a standing soleus stretch (described below) after every hundred steps.

- Vary your gait to promote good range of motion. Try switching between walking on your toes, taking big steps, taking small steps, and walking with your feet turned in and then turned out.

- Walk up stairs or down stairs by approaching the steps at an angle and putting your whole foot onto each step. This technique is also helpful on a ladder or when ascending or descending a steep hill.

- When hiking uphill, take breaks to stretch the soleus, ankle, and calf in all directions.

- Use cruise control on long car trips and take frequent stretching and walking breaks.

- Anytime you sit for more than a short time, use an angled footrest or place a soft pillow under your toes and the front of your feet to give the backs of your lower legs a mild stretch.

- Whenever you're sitting, make sure the seat bottom isn't pressing into the backs of the thighs, as this will reduce blood flow to the lower legs.

Self-Care Treatment

Here are a few general pointers to keep in mind for all compression techniques and stretches described in this chapter:

- Warm the area prior to treatment, especially when your symptoms are severe.

- When sitting or lying on the floor for any form of self-care (compression, stretching, range of motion exercises), a carpeted surface is ideal; alternatively, you can use an exercise mat.

- Treat both legs, even if you have trigger points in only one leg.

- Refer to the MYO compression illustration and compress all areas indicated by X's. The larger circled X's represent likely spots for trigger points, but the entire muscle requires treatment.

- Never exceed a pain level of 6 on a scale of 0 to 10.

- When applying compression, sustain the compression for up to 30 seconds and repeat at least two or three times, or until there's a noticeable decrease in pain and increase in range of motion.

- Gradually increase the amount of compression as you feel the muscle softening and relaxing. Be aware of how the tissues respond to treatment.

- When stretching, hold the position for two to three normal breaths.

- When a stretch is repeated several times on both sides, alternate sides with each repetition.

- After treatment and stretching, do the range of motion exercises given for the soleus in chapter 16.

Compression Treatment

Treat the entire calf with compression so you don't miss any trigger points. This will also enhance circulation throughout the calf. During much of the treatment, you'll need to press through the gastrocnemius to reach the soleus. When you get about halfway down the lower leg, you'll begin to treat the soleus directly. Note that the inner and outer edges of the soleus peek out from under the sides of the gastrocnemius muscle for most of its length.

Because of the location of the soleus, there aren't many options for how to apply compression. Start by sitting down and running your hands over the backs of your calves. Feel for any spots that are painful or harder or denser than the surrounding tissue. You'll mostly be feeling the gastrocnemius muscle, as it's more superficial and covers almost all of the soleus. It is the gastrocnemius that is critically important to proper knee function. If it has trigger points, it can contribute to your back pain because its dysfunction can cause you to walk differently. This muscle is essential for a clean push-off during gait (Simons 2009). So if it is restricted or harboring trigger points, the gastrocnemius will most certainly benefit from the compression treatment as you treat the soleus.

It's easiest to do soleus compression with a Jacknobber, as it's difficult to get enough leverage by using your hands. Look at the pattern of X's marked on figure 14.6. The larger circled X's represent the most likely places to find trigger points. The smaller X's represent all the areas where you should apply compression treatment. Compress all of these areas on each calf, whether or not they're painful and tender. Apply pressure at 1-inch intervals down the calf in three lines, on the inner, middle, and outer edges of the calf, giving extra compression to painful and tender areas before moving to the next spot. You'll compress about thirty points on each calf, which will take up to 10 minutes for each leg. If a friend can help, have them apply compression in these same spots while you lie face-down.

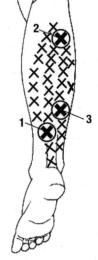

MYO compression for Soleus

Figure 14.6

If these techniques are too painful, try heating the lower leg first using a warm Mother Earth Pillow or Fomentek bag. You can even do compression through a warm Fomentek bag if the pain is severe at first. For less spot-specific compression, try rolling your lower leg over a 5-inch compression therapy ball or a 4- or 6-inch-diameter foam roller while lying face-up on the floor.

You can also apply more spot-specific compression using a stretching strap. This allows you to compress the taut bands while they're stretched, which is more effective unless it's too painful. Place the ball of your foot through one of the loops of the strap and pull your forefoot toward you while resting the back of your calf on a Jacknobber, as shown in figure 14.7. Gradually move your calf to apply compression to the entire surface of the soleus muscle with the Jacknobber, looking for taut bands. Whenever you find a particularly painful or tight spot, maintain the compression until you feel the muscle soften a bit.

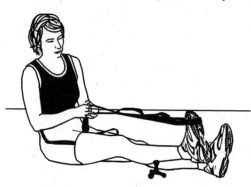

Figure 14.7

Stretching

After applying compression, stretch the soleus. Remember to warm up before stretching. For the soleus, a short walk with variations, such as walking on your toes or walking with your knees bent, or doing the range of motion exercises for the soleus in chapter 16, will provide an effective warm-up.

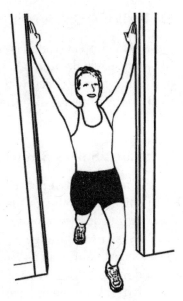

Standing Doorway Stretch

Stand in a doorway and place both hands on the sides of the door-jamb at about shoulder level. Step back about 3 feet with your right foot and put half of your weight on each foot. To stretch the right soleus, bend your left knee, keeping your torso upright and the heel of your right foot on the floor or as close to the floor as possible, as shown in figure 14.8. Gradually increase the stretch by bending your left knee farther and dropping your body toward the floor. Hold this stretch for 15 seconds. Do this stretch at least three times for each leg, and do this twice daily for the first two weeks. Don't stretch beyond a point of mild discomfort, particularly if your lower leg muscles are very tight.

Figure 14.8

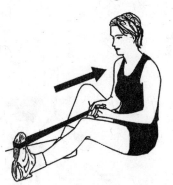

On the Wall Stretch

Sit on the floor with your back against a wall and one leg extended. Wrap a stretching strap or dog leash around the ball of the foot of the extended leg and pull your forefoot toward your knee, as shown in figure 14.9. Increase the intensity gradually until you feel mild discomfort, then gradually decrease it over 10 to 15 seconds. Repeat this stretch at least twice for each leg, and do this twice daily for the first two weeks.

Figure 14.9

Standing Soleus Stretch

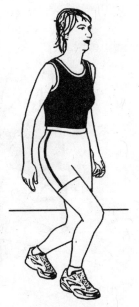

This is one of the easiest and most important stretches for the soleus. You can do it anytime you're standing, or even when walking from one room to another. To eliminate soleus trigger points, you'll need to stretch much more, and much more frequently, than you might think. So we recommend you do this stretch as many as fifteen to twenty times daily, particularly during the first month of self-care treatment.

To stretch the left soleus, start by slightly lunging forward with your right foot and leg. With your left leg behind you, slowly bend your left knee and keep your left heel on the floor, as shown in figure 14.10. Breathe and relax as you hold this stretch for at least 10 seconds. You should feel the stretch in the mid to lower left calf. Do this stretch for both legs, even if you have trigger points only on one side.

Figure 14.10

Walking Up an Incline

Another great stretch is simply walking up an incline. You can do this on a hill, or if you live in the flatlands as we do, find a handicapped ramp and walk up the ramp. As you walk up the incline, stop and bend your back leg with your heel flat on the ramp. Stretch the soleus for two long breaths, and then do the same for the other leg.

Seated Soleus Stretch

As mentioned, repetition of soleus stretches is very important. If you work in a seated position, your soleus naturally gets less activity and less stretching, so we strongly urge you to incorporate the following sequence of seated stretches into your workday.

First sit near the edge of your chair. To stretch your right soleus, extend your right leg and flex your toes toward your head as much as you can, as shown in figure 14.11, and hold for 10 to 15 seconds. You should feel a very distinct stretch in your right calf. Repeat the stretch on the left side.

Next, stretch the opposer muscles in the front of your lower right leg as shown in figure 14.12. In doing this stretch, sit mostly on your left buttock, bend your right knee and straighten your right ankle as much as possible. Hold for 10 to 15 seconds, then repeat on the left side.

Next, stretch the inside of the right ankle as shown in figure 14.13. This stretch helps compensate for the tendency of the soleus to bend the foot inward. Breathe and relax in this position for 10 to 15 seconds, then repeat on the left side.

Finally, stretch the opposers of the soleus muscle by stretching the outside of the ankle as shown in figure 14.14. Again, breathe and relax in this position for at least 10 to 15 seconds.

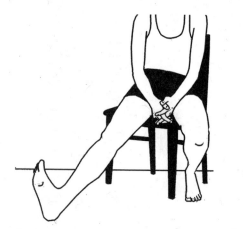

Figure 14.11

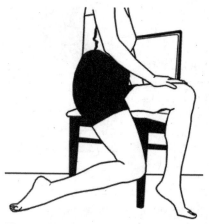

Figure 14.12

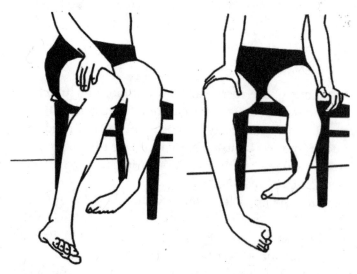

Figure 14.13   Figure 14.14

Contracting and Relaxing

Stretching with Resistance

This exercise is quite similar to stretching in a seated position against a wall, as described above. However, it adds a resistance phase, providing a contraction to increase the benefits of the stretch. Stretching with resistance is particularly useful for correcting soleus dysfunction, which can impair blood circulation, leading to cold feet or swollen ankles, feet, or lower legs. It's also very helpful for soleus trigger points that refer pain to the low back.

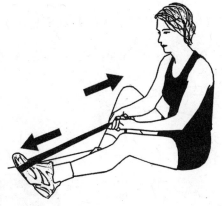

As before, sit with your back against a wall and one leg extended, then place the strap around the ball of the foot of the extended leg. Press your foot down as if to point your toes, using 30 percent of your strength, and resist with the strap, as shown in figure 14.15. Hold for 10 to 15 seconds, then exhale and relax. Next, pull your foot upward toward the knee, flexing the ankle as far as possible without discomfort, as shown in figure 14.9, above. Hold for 10 to 15 seconds, then exhale and relax. Repeat this exercise at least twice for each leg, and do this twice daily for the first two weeks.

Figure 14.15

Moving the Soleus During Normal Activity

Some of the exercises in chapter 16 target the soleus, but this muscle is also easily worked in the course of daily activities. The following simple suggestions allow you to steal time from regular daily activities to help restore full function of your soleus muscles. Think of these as ways to exercise without having to set aside time for it:

- An easy and very important thing to do is to push off your toes when walking. Make sure your feet roll from heels to toes as you walk, finish each step with a gentle but firm push off the toes, and try to keep your feet facing straight forward as you walk. Do this consciously wherever you walk, even just from one room to another.

- When you walk, go a short distance with your feet pointed inward, and then with your feet pointed outward. Exaggerate the toe-in and toe-out positions even if they feel awkward. This helps restore normal range of motion and flexibility to your feet and ankles.

- Try walking backward with your toes in, then out, and then in a neutral position. This may be difficult to do for any considerable distance, but even a small amount of backward walking helps restore full function to the soleus.

- Here's a really easy one! Sit in a rocking chair when watching television or reading. Keep the chair rocking back and forth using both feet, flexing and extending your ankles.

For Practitioners

One of the most important things you can do as a practitioner is to be aware that the soleus muscles can cause chronic low back pain. If you know this and know how to test for and treat dysfunction in this muscle, you'll be light-years ahead of many others in your field.

Assessment and Tests

Palpate the soleus muscle and feel for any unusual contraction or taut bands, especially in the

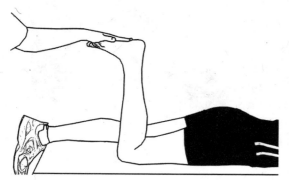

lower third of the posterior lateral calf. Have the patient perform the basic tests found earlier in this chapter, and note any restrictions in the patient's normal range of motion. As you proceed with treatment, improved range of motion indicates progress.

To test for restriction in the soleus, flexor hallucis longus, and flexor digitorum longus, have the patient lie prone with knee bent at a 90-degree angle, as shown in figure 14.16. Dorsiflex the patient's ankle. If the ankle can't flex at least 20 degrees, this indicates abnormal restriction and probably soleus trigger points.

Figure 14.16

Manual Treatment

The soleus can be palpated directly about one-third of the way down the lateral lower leg. Try using thumb compression or a pincer technique. With the patient prone and the knee bent at a right angle, treat the soleus with pincer compression while continually moving the ankle through its range of motion as much as possible, as shown in figures 14.17 and 14.18. Feel for tightness or restriction in the superficial fascia of the lower leg, then press deeper into the soleus.

As an alternative, position the patient on one side and treat the medial border of the leg that's resting on the table and the lateral border of the top leg while it's resting on a bolster or pillow. In order to permanently deactivate soleus trigger points, in some cases it may be necessary to treat other muscles in the lower leg (the synergists and antagonists of the soleus).

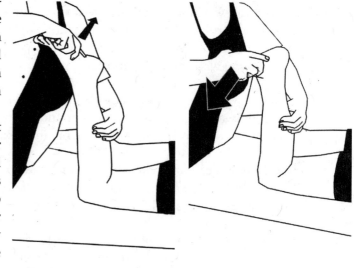

Figure 14.17   Figure 14.18

Spray and Stretch

Here's a spray and stretch technique to ease pain in the back at the sacroiliac joint. As always, be sure to have a source of heat to apply after completing the spray. The lateral soleus trigger point area can refer pain to the low back and buttocks at the sacroiliac joint, trigger point 3 as shown in figure 14.2. Start with the patient standing with hands on the treatment table or on a wall, the right knee bent and the ankle dorsiflexed. The foot should be medially rotated. This position, shown in figure 14.19, creates a maximum stretch of the lateral soleus. Apply the spray upward over the lines shown on the illustration in the direction indicated by the arrows; spraying over trigger point 3 in the lateral soleus. Continue spraying over the thigh and then over the referred pain area at the low back, buttocks, and at the sacroiliac joint. Spray at an acute angle from a distance of approximately 18 inches or more in parallel sweeps. As you spray upward, gently increase the stretch by having the patient further bend the knee, taking up the slack that develops as the soleus releases.

After spraying, immediately apply heat over the area you've sprayed. Then have the patient perform active dorsiflexion and plantar flexion to reestablish full range of motion in the ankle using the pedal series range of motion exercises in the soleus movement protocol in chapter 16.

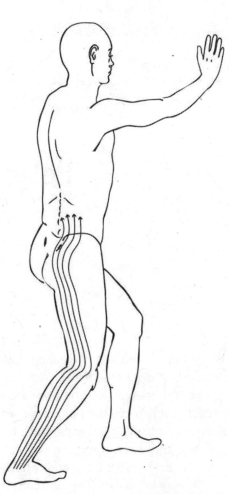

Figure 14.19

Chapter 15

Pelvic Floor Muscles

We can hardly write a book about low back and buttock pain without something about the pelvic floor muscles, which cause what Travell and Simons referred to as that "pain in the rear." It's important to note that pelvic floor pain is often myofascial in origin, contrary to the opinion of many medical experts. And when the pain is caused by muscular dysfunction, the problem is in the muscles of the pelvic floor itself. Long experience tells us that in many cases, pelvic floor pain, as well as pain in the tailbone, the sacrum, and the backs of the thighs, can be alleviated by treating the gluteal muscles, and other muscles in the torso and thighs.

By way of introduction, we can't improve on this quotation from *Clinical Mastery in the Treatment of Myofascial Pain* (Ferguson and Gerwin 2004, 328):

> Chronic pelvic pain is defined as the persistence of unexplained pain in the low abdominal and pelvic tissues without evidence of active disease. This actually is a very vague definition… Medical assessment of the patient complaining of chronic pelvic pain will be dictated by the specialty of the practitioner. The urologist will evaluate the lower urinary tract, and the gynecologist will evaluate the female reproductive organs; the gastroenterologist and colorectal surgeon will evaluate the lower digestive tract. Of course, the orthopaedic physician will look for a skeletal source of the pain. When these medical disciplines can find no pathological conditions, as the definition dictates, they defer to psychiatry. Because there is no diagnostic evidence of an active disease process, the pain has to be "in your head." The common denominator, totally overlooked by most medical practitioners when evaluating a complaint of chronic pelvic pain, is the myofascial component.

This paragraph is amusing if you stand back from it a bit: Imagine these myopic physicians looking only at what they're trained to see and therefore seizing the tail of an elephant and pronouncing it a snake. However, if you suffer from chronic pelvic pain, or pain in the tailbone, the sacrum, or backs of the thighs, it isn't funny—it's sad.

At times, because of the persistence and severity of chronic pelvic pain and the failure of other approaches to treating it, a surgical remedy is attempted, sometimes going to the extreme of removing the bladder, uterus, ovaries, or fallopian tubes. We're not aware of reliable research demonstrating the efficacy of these techniques. In fact, one of the more ironic aspects of chronic pelvic pain is that sometimes the precipitating factor is prolonged positioning of female patients in a physician's stirrups for examination or surgical procedures.

A few years ago, we attended the annual conference of the International Myopain Society, where the keynote speech was given by a German gynecologist. One of his main points touched on the frequency of needless pelvic surgery performed to resolve chronic pain problems that were largely myofascial in origin. Fortunately, we can suggest more practical and less invasive ways to deal with this pain if you suffer from it.

Where Are the Pelvic Floor Muscles and What Do They Do?

The pelvic floor muscles include a bewildering variety of small muscles that together provide a "sling" or "hammock" to support the internal digestive and reproductive organs within the abdominal cavity. In addition to providing a floor for the bottom of the trunk, these muscles help perform the bodily functions of defecation, urination, and sexual intercourse.

The principal muscles of the pelvic floor include the levator ani, sphincter ani, coccygeus, transversus perinei profundus and superficialis, bulbospongiosus, and ischiocavernosus. (Don't worry; there won't be a spelling test.) In addition to the suggestions we offer in this chapter, you can find more extensive treatment recommendations for these muscles in *Myofascial Pain and Dysfunction: The Trigger Point Manual: Upper Half of the Body, Volume 1* (Travell and Simons 1999), chapter 6.

Pelvic Floor Muscle Pain Referral Patterns

Travell and Simons identify six trigger point regions in the pelvic floor muscles, which refer pain to the base of the spine and the back of the thighs. These trigger points can also refer pain to the vagina or the base of the penis. As important, trigger points in the buttock muscles (including the piriformis), the thighs, the lower legs, the back, and the abdomen can all refer pain *to* the pelvic floor region. So active trigger points in these muscles can not only cause pain in the pelvic floor, they can also cause trigger points to develop in the pelvic floor muscles.

What Aggravates the Pelvic Floor Muscles?

In our opinion, the pelvic floor muscles may be the least understood of all the muscles covered in this book. Because pain in the pelvic floor isn't as common as pain in the low back and buttocks, it may not have been the focus of as much research. Based on our clinical experience, here are some of the most likely causes of trigger point activation in the pelvic floor muscles:

- Sitting slumped backward, with the coccyx resting directly on the seat

- Chronic hemorrhoids, inflammation in the pelvic region, or pelvic diseases

- Dysfunction or misalignment of the sacroiliac joint, where the sacrum joins the pelvis

- A severe fall or an accident involving a sudden impact

- Pelvic surgery or even prolonged or frequent vaginal examinations

- Trigger points in one or more of the muscles that refer pain to the pelvic floor

Do I Have Trigger Points in My Pelvic Floor Muscles?

To determine whether you have trigger points in your pelvic floor muscles, first consider the medical evidence. If you have pain in this region but no indication of disease, infection, or structural problems, or if your physician surmises the pain is "all in your head," you can reasonably infer that the pain is likely to be myofascial in origin, with one important qualification: While we don't ever suppose this pain is imaginary, it can at times have psychological origins. Chronic psychological tension can lead to an inability to relax the pelvic floor muscles, and this can activate trigger points.

That said, myofascial causes of this pain are commonly ignored by most physicians, regardless of their training or special expertise. In fact, some specialist physicians are so entrenched in their views that they refuse to refer a patient for examination and treatment by a physical therapist, even when they can find nothing wrong with the patient from their own rather specialized perspective.

After considering the medical evidence, think about the kinds of symptoms you're experiencing. The following symptoms can sometimes help you confirm the presence of trigger points in the pelvic floor (Travell and Simons 1992):

- Intense, burning vaginal pain

- Sharp burning sensations during intercourse

- Deep soreness after intercourse

- Intense pain during or after urination, or a sense of constantly needing to urinate

- Occasional incontinence

- Persistent pain in the lower abdomen, groin, and inner thighs

Because many of these problems fall within the purview of specialist physicians, you may be offered the option of exploratory surgery, even if there's no clear diagnostic basis for it. At the very least, it would be wise to rule out myofascial causes before pursuing that option.

One way to confirm the presence of active trigger points in the pelvic floor muscles is to consult a physical therapist specifically accredited to do intrapelvic examination and treatment. Only a small subset of physical therapists are trained and accredited to do this work, but if you can find one, they can be a good resource. Please be aware that not just any physical therapist will do; most are neither trained nor qualified to deal with this somewhat specialized physical problem. Even some physical therapists who are trained to treat pelvic floor pain may be unfamiliar with the phenomenon of referred pain and therefore be unaware that other muscles could be contributing to chronic pelvic pain.

Another possibility is to treat the muscles that refer pain to the pelvic floor (listed below). Seven of these muscles aren't covered in this book. We suggest you start by treating the eleven muscles that are covered in this book. If the pain in your pelvic floor is reduced or eliminated, you're clearly on the right track. If that doesn't resolve the problem, you'll have to research and treat the other seven muscles or find a practitioner trained to treat them by means of myofascial trigger point techniques.

Possible Referring Muscles Included in This Book	Possible Referring Muscles Not Included in This Book
• Gluteus maximus	• Adductor magnus
• Gluteus medius	• Adductor brevis
• Gluteus minimus	• Gracilis
• Hamstrings (semitendinosus, semimembranosus, and biceps femoris)	• Oblique abdominals
	• Pectineus
• Piriformis	• Sartorius
• Multifidi (see chapter 6, Paraspinals)	• Vastus lateralis
• Iliopsoas	
• Quadratus lumborum	
• Rectus abdominis	
• Soleus	

Many of these muscles attach to parts of the pelvic floor, so it's hardly surprising that chronic activation of trigger points in these muscles can cause pain in the pelvic floor. For example, the gracilis is the long, thin muscle that sticks out from the groin area like a sharp edge when you spread your legs. This muscle is the locus of what is known in the sports world as a "groin pull," which is sometimes felt most severely in and around the pelvic floor. If treating one or more of these muscles reduces or eliminates the pain, you've solved the problem and spared yourself an agonizing journey through several medical subspecialties and possible surgery.

If you treat all the muscles that refer pain to the pelvic floor and the pain persists, the next step is to look for trigger points in the pelvic floor muscles themselves.

Self-Care Treatment

There are no objective tests for trigger points in the pelvic floor muscles. Accordingly, you must deduce this problem by directly palpating the muscles in the pelvic floor. In effect, you're going to test and treat at the same time. In our clinic, we're constantly evaluating tissue as we treat it and noticing how it responds to treatment; here you'll be doing the same thing for yourself. If you treat the pelvic floor area and the pain goes away, you can be certain the problem was myofascial trigger points.

Since we cover treatment of eleven muscles that can refer pain to the pelvic floor in other chapters, we won't repeat any of those treatment techniques in this chapter. Here we're concerned only with treatment of the pelvic floor muscles themselves. We confine our recommendations to various methods of compression which necessarily involve some degree of stretching. If these methods provide partial but not complete relief of your pelvic pain, you might want to consult a physical therapist or other medical practitioner specifically trained to treat this area.

Compression

Pelvic floor pain, as well as pain in the tailbone, the sacrum, and the backs of the thighs, can sometimes be very severe. Accordingly, we urge you to start with gentle compression and go on to firmer and more spot-specific methods as the pain begins to abate.

Using Warm Fomentek Bags and Mother Earth Pillows

First, warm up and relax the muscles for a few minutes by sitting on a warm Fomentek bag on a well-padded chair with armrests. The armrests are important, as they allow you to adjust the pressure on your pelvic floor while sitting in the chair. Next, heat a small Mother Earth Pillow in the microwave, fold it in half, and place it on the chair seat beneath your pelvic floor, between your tailbone and reproductive organs. Tilt your pelvis slowly front to back and then side to side over the pillow. If this causes the pain to abate somewhat, it's likely that you're relaxing and releasing taut bands and trigger points in the pelvic floor muscles.

Using a Tennis Ball

Next, look for trigger points using a tennis ball. It's best to have a somewhat firmer seat for this method, or the ball may sink too far into the chair seat. The armrests are still important because they permit you to control the pressure being applied to the pelvic floor. Place the tennis ball directly between your thighs and just in front of your anus. Lower your pelvis slowly onto the ball, supporting your weight with your arms, and roll slowly from side to side. If this compression causes pain similar to what you regularly experience, you may have found the source of your pain. Continue to compress the areas that are particularly sensitive, making sure not to go beyond a pain level of 6 on a scale of 0 to 10. If the pressure is too much, try using a soft, thin cushion or a warm Fomentek bag on the chair seat with the tennis ball beneath it.

Using the Backnobber

Next, you can look for trigger points in the pelvic region using a Backnobber. Place the larger part of the tool under your pelvis as you remain seated on a well-padded chair. Press gently forward on the upper end of the tool so that the knob beneath you presses into your pelvic floor just forward of the anus and toward either of the sit bones. Gradually and carefully adjust the position of the tool so you compress different areas of the pelvic floor. When you find a painful spot, stay on it and gradually increase the pressure for about 10 seconds, then gradually release it.

Once you've reduced the pain somewhat with one or both of the first two methods of compression, the Backnobber will probably be the most effective tool for applying compression to this muscle group. Once you become familiar with how to use it, it offers an unparalleled degree of leverage and control.

For Practitioners

We can't add specific instructions for practitioners beyond what we've said above. However, we can reiterate how important it is for you to be aware that chronic pelvic pain very often has a myofascial origin. Because so few practitioners are aware of this, chronic pelvic pain usually ends up in the hands of specialists, who tend to look for causes pertaining to their particular area of expertise. When they don't find such causes, they often dismiss the pain as being unimportant or psychological in origin, or they refer to another specialist. We don't propose that pelvic floor pain is always myofascial in origin, merely that it often is. So we urge you to read this entire chapter if you encounter patients with pelvic floor pain. We believe this will help you properly evaluate these patients and advise them on how to treat the myofascial component when it is present.

Chapter 16

Range of Motion Exercises

Movement through the full nonpainful range of motion is one of the four components of self-care. (As a reminder, the other three are warming up, compression, and sequences of stretching, contracting, and relaxing.) Range of motion exercise is distinct from stretching and contraction, although it contains elements of both. We end all treatments with stretching and then usually three repetitions of nonpainful range of motion exercise. We also use range of motion exercise to prevent trigger points from recurring and to prevent new trigger points from occurring.

Many people find that their muscles are short, tight, and painful when they wake up in the morning or after long periods of inactivity. Taut bands and trigger points often set in due to inactivity and may result in referred pain and swelling where the muscles attach to the bone. To counteract this, we recommend doing range of motion exercises for any stiff or tight muscles after you get up in the morning or any time you've been inactive for a while. This will train the muscles in full lengthening and full shortening. The inability to fully lengthen often indicates trigger points and taut bands. The inability to shorten causes what we call "pseudo weakness." We use this term because when we eliminate the taut bands and trigger points, the muscle is strong again right away, without any need for strengthening exercises.

With chronic pain conditions, the whole muscle usually needs reeducation. To work all parts of the muscle, it's often necessary to incorporate variations into the movement. With sufficient variation, all of the muscle fibers will be taken through their range of motion. In addition to changing the movement itself, you can introduce variation in many other ways: Change the surface you exercise on, using hard, soft, slanted, or uneven surfaces. Move on sand or move in water, whether knee-high or waist-high. Make the movements larger or smaller, and experiment with making them really, really small and really, really large. Vary the tempo, moving more slowly or more quickly. It can even be helpful to wear two or three different pairs of shoes throughout the day, as long as they're sensible shoes that offer you good support.

Most people need a lot more range of motion exercise than they think they do. Try to integrate range of motion exercise into your daily life as much as possible, focusing on the exercises appropriate for whichever muscles contain trigger points and taut bands. To make this easy for you, we've grouped the exercises into protocols for each of the muscles covered in the book (with one protocol for all three gluteal muscles). Many of the exercises benefit multiple muscles, and each protocol includes a list of other exercises that also benefit that muscle. Whenever possible, do these exercises to music. This will make it a lot more fun, and the speed and feeling of the music will encourage you to incorporate more variations into your movements. If it's fun, you'll do it more, and more is what you need! You can also incorporate many range of motion exercises into other activities, so that you don't always have to set aside time specifically for range of motion exercise. Try to include some range of motion exercise as you walk from one room to another at work or at home.

As you start doing range of motion exercises, it's important to take it easy and go slowly. At first, do the exercises slowly, using small movements and doing just a few reps—perhaps four to eight repetitions. For exercises that have beginning, intermediate, and advanced versions, always start with the beginner version. With time, gradually increase your range of motion and speed and work up to sixteen repetitions or more. Throughout, your movements should be as pain-free as possible. If an exercise is painful, back off, reducing the extent and speed of the motion until you experience little or no pain. Once you feel no pain for several days in a row, you can gradually increase the extent, speed, and number of reps. Likewise, once a beginner version becomes comfortable, you can start working on the next level. For exercises done on the floor, it's best to use a carpeted surface or exercise mat.

In many of the exercises, we describe "tilting of the pelvis" backward or forward. For your reference, we would like to walk you through this movement to better clarify what we mean. Place your hands at your waist and press in and downward. You should be feeling the top of your pelvis, called the iliac crest. Look on page 141, figure 11.1 to see this bony landmark. It is from this top rim that we describe tilting. If it moves forward, then it is considered to be "tilted forward" or anterior pelvic tilt. When it is moved backward, it is called "tilted backward" or posterior pelvic tilt.

Range of Motion Protocol for Iliopsoas

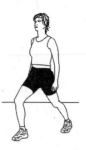

Big Steps

Iliopsoas, hamstrings, soleus, gluteus maximus, gluteus medius, gluteus minimus

While walking, alternate taking normal steps and big steps. Work up to doing a series of 16 big steps. This exercise is easy to do anytime you're walking, throughout your normal daily activities.

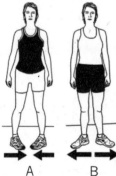

A   B

Standing Hip Twist

Iliopsoas, hamstrings, gluteus medius, gluteus minimus, piriformis, gluteus maximus, soleus

Start with your right foot in front of your left, with both feet pointed outward (A). Accentuate a big hip twist inward, slowly pivoting on the ball of your right foot and rotating your right foot, knee, leg, and hip inward (B). Slowly return to the starting position. Do 4 reps before switching to the other side. Gradually increase the speed and number of reps as you gain mobility.

Standing Toes In and Out

Iliopsoas, hamstrings, gluteus medius, gluteus minimus, piriformis, gluteus maximus, soleus

A   B

Stand for a time with your toes pointed inward (A), then stand with your toes pointed outward (B). Gradually adopting a more extreme inward and outward position over time may seem like a very slight movement, but it's very beneficial for the psoas, the hamstrings, and, especially, the gluteal muscles.

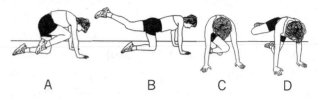

A   B   C   D

All-Fours Series

Iliopsoas, hamstrings, gluteus maximus, gluteus medius, gluteus minimus, piriformis

From an all-fours position, bring your right knee to your chest (A), then swing your right leg back and up (B). Swing your right knee forward again, but this time across your chest toward your left elbow (C). Bring your right leg out to the side and up to about hip level, keeping the knee bent (D). Bring your right leg back down to the starting position. At first, alternate legs with each repetition. As you gain strength and flexibility, do multiple reps with each leg before switching to the other leg.

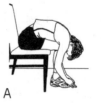

A

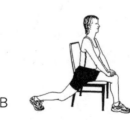

B

Seated Flex and Extension

Iliopsoas, rectus abdominis, gluteus maximus, soleus

Start in a chair with no armrests and sit near the right edge of the chair seat. Relax your abs and slowly lower your chest to your thighs, letting your hands touch the floor (A). As you begin to come back to an upright position, extend your right leg behind you as far as you can without pain (B). Try to keep your hips and abs as relaxed as possible. Do 4 reps on the right side, then repeat the sequence on the left.

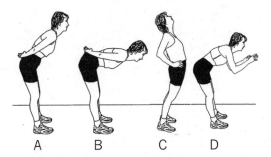

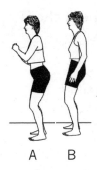

Standing Pelvic Tilt

Iliopsoas, rectus abdominis, paraspinals, hamstrings, gluteus maximus, quadratus lumborum, soleus

Stand with your knees bent. Inhale, relax your abdominals, and slowly tilt your pelvis forward (A). Return to the starting position, then exhale and pull your abdominals in as you slowly tilt your pelvis backward (B). You can also do pelvic tilts while walking: Just walk for a short distance, stop, do a series of four pelvic tilts, and then resume walking. You can repeat this as many times as you like—more is better.

Torso Bend and Extend Series

Iliopsoas, rectus abdominis, hamstrings, paraspinals, gluteus maximus, soleus, quadratus lumborum

Beginner: Stand with your knees straight and your hands behind your back. Slowly bend forward at your hips with your back straight (A), bending as far as you can without pain. Slowly return to the starting position. Over time, bend farther until you can achieve a 90-degree forward bend (B). After returning to the starting position, place your hands on your hips, then slowly and gently extend your torso backward (C). Start small, arching back as little as 5 degrees at first. Slowly return to a neutral position and relax all of the muscles in your back and torso. Gradually work up to as much as 20 or 30 degrees of pain-free torso extension.

Intermediate: Stand with your arms up, elbows bent, with your hands in front of your face. Slowly bend forward at your hips with your back straight (D), bending as far as you can without pain. Slowly return to the starting position. Over time, bend farther until you can achieve a 90-degree forward bend. After returning to the starting position, keep your hands and arms in the same position and slowly and gently extend your torso backward. Start small, arching back as little as 5 degrees at first. Slowly return to a neutral position and relax all of the muscles in your back and torso. Gradually work up to as much as 20 or 30 degrees of pain-free torso extension.

Advanced: Stand with both arms extended overhead. Slowly bend forward at your hips with your back straight. Bend as far as you can without pain. Slowly return to the starting position. Over time, bend farther until you can achieve a 90-degree forward bend. After returning to the starting position, keep your arms overhead and slowly and gently extend your torso backward. Slowly return to a neutral position and relax all of the muscles in your back and torso. Again, start small and work your way up to greater extension with time.

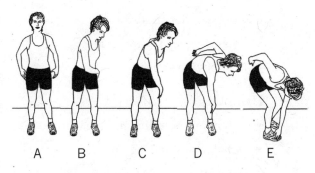

Standing Twist and Bend Series

Iliopsoas, rectus abdominis, paraspinals, gluteus maximus, gluteus medius, gluteus minimus, hamstrings, soleus, quadratus lumborum

Begin in a standing position, with your hands at your sides (A). Twist your torso and touch your right hand to your left hip (B), then return to the starting position. Twist a bit farther and bring your right hand to your left thigh (C), then return to the starting position. Repeat, this time reaching a bit farther down your left leg (D), then return to the starting position. Finally, if you can do so without pain, reach all the way down to your left foot (E). Repeat the entire sequence on the opposite side.

Other exercises that will benefit the iliopsoas

- Rectus abdominis protocol
    - Seated pelvic tilt
    - Seated pelvic tilt on a fitness ball

- Quadratus lumborum protocol
    - Standing hip swing
    - Standing hip hike
    - Fitness ball side stretch
    - Standing side stretch
    - Standing side bend

- Gluteal muscles protocol
    - Standing leg swing series
    - Grapevine series

- Hamstrings protocol
    - Dynamic standing and bending
    - Dynamic standing on one leg

- Soleus protocol
    - Walking uphill

Range of Motion Protocol for Paraspinals

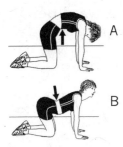

Cat Back and Old Horse

Paraspinals, rectus abdominis, quadratus lumborum, gluteus maximus

Starting on all fours, exhale and slowly lift your mid-torso toward the ceiling like a cat arching its back (A). Hold for at least 5 seconds, then inhale and slowly lower your mid-torso toward the floor like an old, swayback horse, relaxing your abdominals and lifting your head and buttocks (B). Hold for at least 5 seconds.

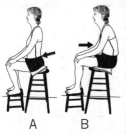

Seated Pelvic Tilt

Paraspinals, gluteus maximus, rectus abdominis, iliopsoas, quadratus lumborum

Sit on a chair or high stool topped with a dynamic surface, such as a Fomentek bag or an air-filled seating disk, with your feet on the ground, or sit on a stool with your feet on a footstool. Inhale, relax your abdominals, and slowly tilt the top of your pelvis forward (A), creating a slight arch in your back. Return to the starting position, then exhale and pull your abdominals in as you slowly tilt your pelvis back (B).

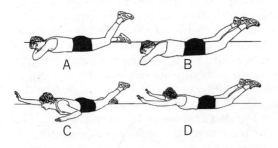

Superman

Paraspinals, gluteus maximus, gluteus medius, gluteus minimus, hamstrings, quadratus lumborum

Beginner: Start by lying on the floor face-down, with your arms folded in front of you and your head resting on your arms. Slowly raise your left leg toward the ceiling (A). Hold for 5 seconds, then slowly lower the leg to the floor. Relax, then repeat with your right leg.

Intermediate: Starting in the same position, slowly raise both legs toward the ceiling (B). Hold for 5 seconds, then slowly lower both legs to the floor.

Advanced: Start by lying on the floor face-down, with your arms fully extended as if you were flying like Superman. Slowly raise your left leg and right arm and head toward the ceiling (C). Hold for 5 seconds, then slowly lower them to the floor. Relax, then repeat with your right leg, left arm, and head. Hold for 5 seconds, then slowly lower them to the floor. Relax, then slowly raise both arms, both legs, and your head simultaneously (D). Hold for 5 seconds, then slowly return to the starting position. If you can do this for several reps, you are definitely a superman or superwoman! Remember, don't do this movement unless you can do it without inducing pain.

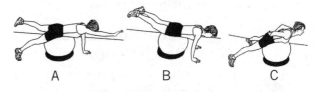

Prone Fitness Ball Series

Paraspinals, gluteus maximus, hamstrings, quadratus lumborum

Beginner: This exercise isn't recommended for beginners.

Intermediate: Use a large fitness ball with a base for stability. Lie face-down across the ball with the ball under the center of your body and your hands and feet on the floor for support. Slowly raise your right arm and left leg (A). Hold for 4 seconds, then slowly lower them to the floor. Relax, then repeat with your left arm and right leg.

Advanced: Starting in the same position, shift your weight onto your hands, contract your gluteal muscles, and slowly raise your legs upward (B). Hold for 3 seconds, then slowly return to the starting position. Next, shift your weight onto your feet, place your hands on your lower back, and slowly raise your torso upward using your back muscles (C). Hold for 3 seconds, then slowly return to the starting position. If necessary, anchor one or both feet along a baseboard as you do this exercise.

Range of Motion Protocol for Paraspinals

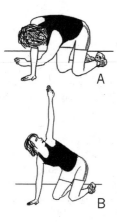

Thread the Needle

Paraspinals, rectus abdominis, quadratus lumborum

Starting on all fours, reach your left arm through to the right under your chest (A), rotating your head, neck, and torso to the right and following your hand with your eyes. Bring your left arm slowly back through the "needle" and then up toward the ceiling (B), rotating your head, neck, and torso to the left and following your hand with your eyes. Repeat on the other side. For a more advanced version, use a very light weight (1 or 2 pounds) in the moving hand.

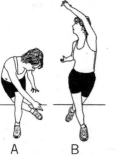

Torso Rotation and Reach Series

Paraspinals, quadratus lumborum, gluteus medius, gluteus maximus

Beginner: Start small and gradually extend the movements as you become more flexible. From a standing position, step your right leg back, crossing it behind your left foot (A) and keeping most of your weight on your left leg. Simultaneously, reach across your torso with your right arm, bringing it down and across your left thigh, and allow your left arm to swing back. Return to the starting position, then step forward with your right leg, twist your torso to the right, and swing both arms to the right, your right arm behind and your left arm up (B).

Intermediate: To take it up a notch, simply take larger steps and reach your arms farther.

Advanced: For the most advanced movement, take even larger steps, reach your front hand down to the floor in the first half of the motion, and twist your torso farther around in the second half of the motion.

Seated Forward Bend

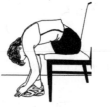

Paraspinals, gluteus maximus

Sit upright in a chair, then slowly bend forward while keeping your abdominal and thigh muscles relaxed. Rest your chest on your thighs and take a deep breath. Return slowly to the starting position.

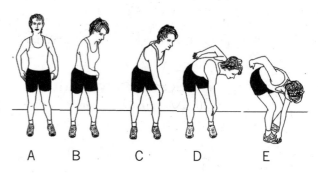

Standing Twist and Bend Series

Paraspinals, rectus abdominis, iliopsoas, hamstrings, quadratus lumborum, gluteus medius, gluteus maximus, gluteus minimus, soleus

Begin in a standing position, with your hands at your sides (A). Twist your torso and touch your right hand to your left hip (B), then return to the starting position. Twist a bit farther and bring your right hand to your left thigh (C), then return to the starting position. Repeat, this time reaching a bit farther down your left leg (D), then return to the starting position. Finally, if you can do so without pain, reach all the way down to your left foot (E). Repeat the entire sequence on the opposite side. To add a greater stretch to the muscles in front and a greater contraction to the muscles in back, lift the moving arm up and back each time you return to the starting position.

Other exercises that will benefit the paraspinals

- Iliopsoas protocol
  - Torso bend and extend series

- Rectus abdominis protocol
  - Standing pelvic tilt
  - Seated pelvic tilt on a fitness ball

- Quadratus lumborum protocol
  - Seated back twist
  - Fitness ball side stretch
  - Standing twist
  - Standing side stretch
  - Standing side bend

- Gluteal muscles protocol
  - Dynamic standing on one leg

- Piriformis protocol
  - Standing leg swing adaptation

- Hamstrings protocol
  - Forward torso bend series
  - Dynamic standing and bending
  - Dynamic standing on one leg

- Soleus protocol
  - Knee bend series

Range of Motion Protocol for Rectus Abdominis

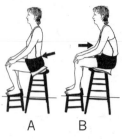

Seated Pelvic Tilt

Rectus abdominis, paraspinals, gluteus maximus, iliopsoas, quadratus lumborum

Sit in a chair or stool on a dynamic surface, such as a Fomentek bag or an air-filled seating disk, with your feet on the ground, or sit on a stool with your feet on a footstool. Inhale, relax your abdominals, and slowly tilt your pelvis forward (A), creating a slight arch in your back. Return to the starting position, then exhale as you slowly tilt your pelvis back (B).

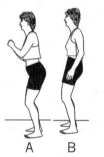

Standing Pelvic Tilt

Rectus abdominis, paraspinals, gluteus maximus, iliopsoas, hamstrings, quadratus lumborum, soleus

Stand with your knees bent. Inhale, relax your abdominals, and slowly tilt your pelvis forward (A). Return to the starting position, then exhale and slowly tilt your pelvis back (B). You can also do pelvic tilts while walking: Just walk for a short distance, stop, do a series of 4 pelvic tilts, and then resume walking. You can repeat this as many times as you like—more is better.

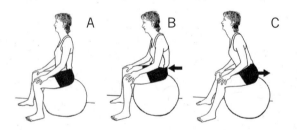

Seated Pelvic Tilt on a Fitness Ball

Rectus abdominis, paraspinals, quadratus lumborum, gluteus maximus, gluteus minimus

Sit on the front half of a large fitness ball with your feet spread for stability (A). Do seated pelvic tilts as described above, rolling slightly on the ball as you tilt back and curl forward. Exhale and contract your abs as you bring your pubic bone up toward your belly button (B). As you inhale, relax your abdominals and allow your belly to stick out as you slightly arch your low back (C), then return to the starting position.

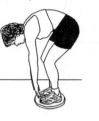

Dynamic Standing and Bending

Rectus abdominis, paraspinals, gluteus maximus, gluteus medius, gluteus minimus, quadratus lumborum, hamstrings, soleus, iliopsoas

Stand balanced on both feet on a surface that will be wobbly when you stand on it, like a dynamic seating disk partially filled with air, a balance or wobble board, a piece of dense foam, or a pillow. Exhale and slowly bend forward, slightly bending your knees and keeping your balance as you touch your toes or the floor with your fingertips, keeping your abdominal muscles relaxed. Inhale and slowly straighten your back to return to a standing position. This movement requires good balance. Until you've mastered it, lightly grasp a sturdy chair or other support to help you keep your balance.

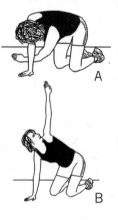

Thread the Needle

Rectus abdominis, paraspinals, quadratus lumborum

Starting on all fours, reach your left arm through to the right under your chest (A), rotating your head, neck, and torso to the right and following your hand with your eyes. Bring your left arm slowly back through the "needle" and then up toward the ceiling (B), rotating your head, neck, and torso to the left and following your hand with your eyes. Repeat on the other side. For a more advanced version, use a very light weight (1 or 2 pounds) in the moving hand.

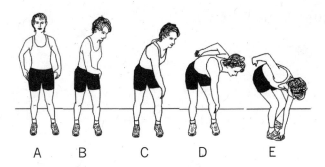

A   B   C   D   E

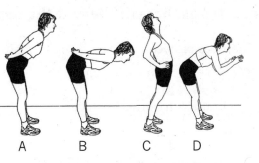

A   B   C   D

Standing Twist and Bend Series

Rectus abdominis, iliopsoas, paraspinals, hamstrings, quadratus lumborum, gluteus maximus, gluteus medius, gluteus minimus, soleus

Begin in a standing position, with your hands at your sides (A). Twist your torso and touch your right hand to your left hip (B), then return to the starting position. Twist a bit farther and bring your right hand to your left thigh (C), then return to the starting position. Repeat, this time reaching a bit farther down your left leg (D), then return to the starting position. Finally, if you can do so without pain, reach all the way down to your left foot (E). Repeat the entire sequence on the opposite side.

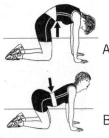

Cat Back and Old Horse

Rectus abdominis, paraspinals, quadratus lumborum, gluteus maximus

A

B

Starting on all fours, exhale and slowly lift your mid-torso toward the ceiling like a cat arching its back (A). Hold for at least 5 seconds, then inhale and slowly lower your mid-torso toward the floor like an old horse, relaxing your abdominals and lifting your head and buttocks (B). Hold for at least 5 seconds.

Torso Bend and Extend Series

Rectus abdominis, hamstrings, paraspinals, gluteus maximus, soleus, iliopsoas, quadratus lumborum

Beginner: Stand with your knees straight and your hands behind your back. Slowly bend forward at your hips with your back straight (A), bending as far as you can without pain. Slowly return to the starting position. Over time, bend farther until you can achieve a 90-degree forward bend (B). After returning to the starting position, place your hands on your hips, then slowly and gently extend your torso backward (C). Start small, arching back as little as 5 degrees at first. Slowly return to a neutral position and relax all of the muscles in your back and torso. Gradually work up to as much as 20 or 30 degrees of pain-free torso extension.

Intermediate: Stand with your arms up, elbows bent, with your hands in front of your face. Slowly bend forward at your hips with your back straight (D), bending as far as you can without pain. Slowly return to the starting position. Over time, bend farther until you can achieve a 90-degree forward bend. After returning to the starting position, keep your hands and arms in the same position and slowly and gently extend your torso backward. Start small, arching back as little as 5 degrees at first. Slowly return to a neutral position and relax all of the muscles in your back and torso. Gradually work up to as much as 20 or 30 degrees of pain-free torso extension.

Advanced: Stand with both arms extended overhead. Slowly bend forward at your hips with your back straight. Bend as far as you can without pain. Slowly return to the starting position. Over time, bend farther until you can achieve a 90-degree forward bend. After returning to the starting position, keep your arms overhead and slowly and gently extend your torso backward. Slowly return to a neutral position and relax all of the muscles in your back and torso. Again, start small and work your way up to greater extension with time.

Other exercises that will benefit the rectus abdominis

- Iliopsoas protocol
  - Seated flex and extension

- Quadratus lumborum protocol
  - Standing hip swing
  - Standing hip hike
  - Seated back twist
  - Fitness ball side stretch
  - Standing side stretch
  - Standing side bend

- Hamstrings protocol
  - Dynamic standing and bending

Range of Motion Protocol for Quadratus Lumborum

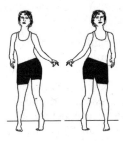

Standing Hip Swing

Quadratus lumborum, iliopsoas, rectus abdominis, soleus

While standing, swing your hips from side to side, keeping your shoulders and chest in a fixed position.

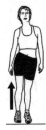

Standing Hip Hike

Quadratus lumborum, iliopsoas, rectus abdominis, soleus

While standing, raise your right hip up, then push it down. Do up to 10 repetitions on the right side, then repeat on the left.

Seated Back Twist

Quadratus lumborum, paraspinals, rectus abdominis

Sit on a stool and, keeping your hips and legs facing straight forward, exhale and twist your upper body to one side as far as you can without pain, leading with the shoulder and arm on the side you're twisting toward. After a count of 2, inhale deeply as you return to the neutral position. Repeat on the other side.

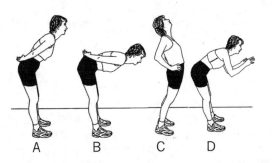

A   B   C   D

Torso Bend and Extend Series

Quadratus lumborum, rectus abdominis, hamstrings, paraspinals, gluteus maximus, soleus, iliopsoas

Beginner: Stand with your knees straight and your hands behind your back. Slowly bend forward at your hips with your back straight (A), bending as far as you can without pain. Slowly return to the starting position. Over time, bend farther until you can achieve a 90-degree forward bend (B). After returning to the starting position, place your hands on your hips, then slowly and gently extend your torso backward (C). Start small, arching back as little as 5 degrees at first. Slowly return to a neutral position and relax all of the muscles in your back and torso. Gradually work up to as much as 20 or 30 degrees of pain-free torso extension.

Intermediate: Stand with your arms up, elbows bent, with your hands in front of your face. Slowly bend forward at your hips with your back straight (D), bending as far as you can without pain. Slowly return to the starting position. Over time, bend farther until you can achieve a 90-degree forward bend. After returning to the starting position, keep your hands and arms in the same position and slowly and gently extend your torso backward. Start small, arching back as little as 5 degrees at first. Slowly return to a neutral position and relax all of the muscles in your back and torso. Gradually work up to as much as 20 or 30 degrees of pain-free torso extension.

Advanced: Stand with both arms extended overhead. Slowly bend forward at your hips with your back straight. Bend as far as you can without pain. Slowly return to the starting position. Over time, bend farther until you can achieve a 90-degree forward bend. After returning to the starting position, keep your arms overhead and slowly and gently extend your torso backward. Slowly return to a neutral position and relax all of the muscles in your back and torso. Again, start small and work your way up to greater extension with time.

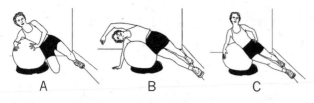

Fitness Ball Side Stretch

Quadratus lumborum, paraspinals, iliopsoas, rectus abdominis

This exercise isn't recommended for beginners; try it only if you have good overall fitness and little or no pain. Kneel down on your right knee, anchor your left foot against a baseboard, and lean sideways over a large fitness ball (A). (At first, it's safer to use a fitness ball with a base, for stability. As you gain strength and balance, you can try it without the base.) Arch your body sideways over the ball and stretch your left arm over your head, bracing yourself against the baseboard with both feet and using your right arm to brace yourself on the floor (B). Lower your left arm to your side and raise your torso up (C). Start with just a few reps and increase with time and practice. Repeat the entire sequence on the other side.

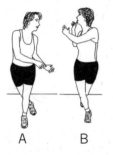

Standing Twist

Quadratus lumborum, paraspinals, gluteus maximus, gluteus medius, gluteus minimus, hamstrings, soleus

From a standing position with your arms by your sides, step back with your right leg and swing your arms to the left as far as you comfortably can (A). Return to the starting position, then repeat on the other side (B). As you repeat this movement, vary the level of your arm swings each time.

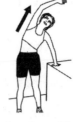

Standing Side Stretch

Quadratus lumborum, iliopsoas, rectus abdominis, paraspinals, soleus

Stand to the right of a table with your legs shoulder width apart. Place your left hand on the table, raise your right arm over your head, and lean over the table, reaching to the left with your right arm. This stretches your waist muscles on the right side and contracts the waist muscles on your left side. Next, bend your left elbow and bring it down to your hip, deepening the stretch and contraction. Slowly return to a neutral standing position, then turn around and repeat the movement on the other side.

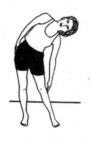

Standing Side Bend

Quadratus lumborum, paraspinals, iliopsoas, rectus abdominis, soleus

Stand with your legs shoulder width apart and your arms at your sides. Relax your abdominal and back muscles and bend over to the left as far as you can without pain, stretching your waist on the right and contracting it on the left. Hold this position for a count of 2, then stand up straight for a count of 2. Repeat on the other side.

Other exercises that will benefit the quadratus lumborum

- Paraspinals protocol
  - Cat back and old horse
  - Superman
  - Prone fitness ball series
  - Thread the needle
  - Torso rotation and reach series
  - Standing twist and bend series

- Rectus abdominis protocol
  - Seated pelvic tilt
  - Standing pelvic tilt
  - Seated pelvic tilt on a fitness ball
  - Dynamic standing and bending

- Gluteal muscles protocol
  - Standing leg swing series
  - Grapevine series

Range of Motion Protocol for Gluteal Muscles

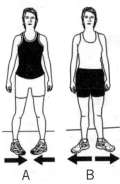

Standing Toes In and Out

Gluteus medius, gluteus minimus, gluteus maximus, iliopsoas, hamstrings, piriformis, soleus

Stand for a time with your toes pointed inward (A), then stand with your toes pointed outward (B). Gradually adopting a more extreme inward and outward position over time may seem like a very slight movement, but it's very beneficial for the psoas, the hamstrings, and, especially, the gluteal muscles.

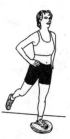

Dynamic Standing on One Leg

Gluteus maximus, hamstrings, soleus, paraspinals, iliopsoas

Beginner: It's best to work up to this standing on one leg on a dynamic surface by first practicing standing on one leg on a regular floor. Once you can do that for one minute, move up to the intermediate level.

Intermediate: Stand balanced on one foot on a surface that will be wobbly when you stand on it, like a dynamic seating disk partially filled with air, a balance or wobble board, a piece of dense foam, or a pillow. Start by trying to balance for 10 seconds, and increase the length of time as you progress. Until you've really mastered this movement, lightly grasp a sturdy chair or table to help maintain your balance. Repeat on the other side.

Advanced: While standing and balancing on one foot on a dynamic surface as described above, slowly bend down toward the floor, then return to an upright position. If you're really good at this, you can try picking up a light weight from the floor.

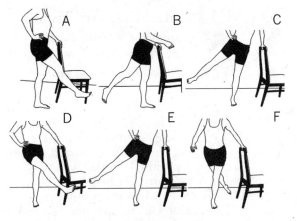

Standing Leg Swing Series

Gluteus maximus, gluteus medius, gluteus minimus, piriformis, iliopsoas, hamstrings, quadratus lumborum, soleus

To help you balance throughout this series, lightly grasp a sturdy chair or countertop with your left hand. Standing behind and to the right of the chair with your right arm on your hip or at your side, swing your right leg forward (A), and then back (B). Turn 90 degrees to your right, then swing your right leg out to the right side (C), and then across to the left in front of your body (D). Swing it out to the right side again (E), and then across behind your body (F). Repeat on the other side. Do as many as 8 reps (work up to this number over time) before switching to the other side.

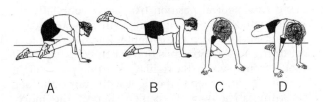

All-Fours Series

Gluteus maximus, gluteus medius, gluteus minimus, iliopsoas, hamstrings, piriformis

From an all-fours position, bring your right knee to your chest (A), then swing your right leg back and up (B). Swing your right knee forward again, but this time across your chest toward your left elbow (C). Bring your right leg out to the side and up to about hip level, keeping the knee bent (D). Bring your right leg back down to the starting position. At first, alternate legs with each repetition. As you gain strength and flexibility, do multiple reps with each leg before switching to the other leg.

Range of Motion Protocol for Gluteal Muscles

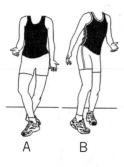

Standing Hip Twist

Gluteus maximus, gluteus medius, gluteus minimus, iliopsoas, hamstrings, piriformis, soleus

Start with your right foot in front of your left, with both feet pointed outward (A). Accentuate a big hip twist inward, slowly pivoting on the ball of your right foot and rotating your right foot, knee, leg, and hip inward (B). Slowly return to the starting position. Do 4 reps before switching to the other side. Gradually increase the speed and number of reps as you gain mobility.

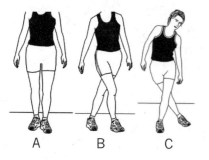

Grapevine Series

Gluteus maximus, gluteus medius, gluteus minimus, quadratus lumborum, iliopsoas, hamstrings, soleus

Stand in a neutral position (A). Cross your left foot behind you and to the right (B), shifting your weight to your left foot. Step to the right with your right foot, returning to a neutral position. Then cross your left foot in front of you to the right (C), shifting your weight to your left foot. Step to the right with your right foot, returning to a neutral position. Repeat the movement, alternating crossing behind and in front with the left foot for 10 to 12 yards, always stepping to the right. Repeat the same sequence in the opposite direction, crossing your right foot first behind and then in front of the left. As you become more familiar with the grapevine, try taking bigger steps.

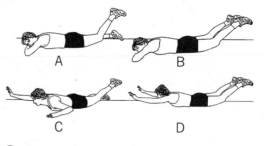

Superman

Gluteus maximus, gluteus medius, gluteus minimus, hamstrings, paraspinals, quadratus lumborum

Beginner: Start by lying on the floor face-down, with your arms folded in front of you and your head resting on your arms. Slowly raise your left leg toward the ceiling (A). Hold for 5 seconds, then slowly lower the leg to the floor. Relax, then repeat with your right leg.

Intermediate: Starting in the same position, slowly raise both legs toward the ceiling (B). Hold for 5 seconds, then slowly lower both legs to the floor.

Advanced: Start by lying on the floor face-down, with your arms fully extended as if you were flying like Superman. Slowly raise your left leg and right arm and head toward the ceiling (C). Hold for 5 seconds, then slowly lower them to the floor. Relax, then repeat with your right leg, left arm, and head. Hold for 5 seconds, then slowly lower them to the floor. Relax, then slowly raise both arms, both legs, and your head simultaneously (D). Hold for 5 seconds, then slowly return to the starting position. If you can do this for several reps, you are definitely a superman or superwoman! Remember, don't do this movement unless you can do it without pain.

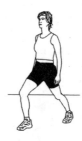

Big Steps

Gluteus maximus, gluteus medius, gluteus minimus, iliopsoas, hamstrings, soleus

While walking, alternate taking normal steps and big steps. Work up to doing a series of 16 big steps. This exercise is easy to do anytime you're walking, throughout your normal daily activities.

Other exercises that will benefit the gluteal muscles

- Iliopsoas protocol
  - Seated flex and extension
  - Torso bend and extend series
  - Standing twist and bend series

- Paraspinals protocol
  - Cat back and old horse
  - Prone fitness ball series
  - Torso rotation and reach series
  - Seated forward bend

- Rectus abdominis protocol
  - Seated pelvic tilt
  - Standing pelvic tilt
  - Seated pelvic tilt on a fitness ball
  - Dynamic standing and bending

- Quadratus lumborum protocol
  - Standing twist

- Piriformis protocol
  - Seated leg cross

- Hamstrings
  - Forward torso bend series

- Soleus protocol
  - Walking uphill
  - Walking uphill with toes in and out
  - Knee bend series

Range of Motion Protocol for Piriformis

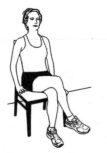

Seated Leg Cross

Piriformis, gluteus medius, gluteus minimus, gluteus maximus

Sit in a chair and cross your right knee completely over your left. Hold for at least 10 seconds, then return to a neutral seated position. Repeat the leg cross on the other side.

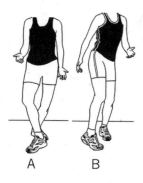

Standing Hip Twist

Piriformis, gluteus medius, gluteus minimus, hamstrings, iliopsoas, gluteus maximus, soleus

Start with your right foot in front of your left, with both feet pointed outward (A). Accentuate a big hip twist inward, slowly pivoting on the ball of your right foot and rotating your right foot, knee, leg, and hip inward (B). Slowly return to the starting position. Do 4 reps before switching to the other side. Gradually increase the speed and number of reps as you gain mobility.

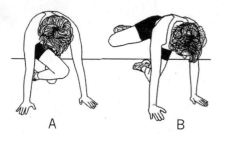

Partial All-Fours Series

Piriformis, iliopsoas, hamstrings, gluteus maximus, gluteus medius, gluteus minimus

From an all-fours position, bring your right knee toward your chest and across toward your left elbow (A). Next, bring your right leg out to the side and up to about hip level, keeping the knee bent (B). At first, alternate legs with each repetition. As you gain strength and flexibility, do multiple reps with each leg before switching to the other leg.

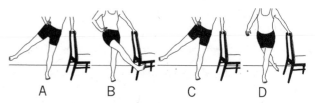

Standing Leg Swing Adaptation

Piriformis, gluteus medius, gluteus minimus, gluteus maximus, iliopsoas, paraspinals, hamstrings, quadratus lumborum, soleus

To help you balance throughout this series, lightly grasp a sturdy chair or countertop with your left hand. Standing with your left hip about a foot behind the back of the chair, swing your right leg out to the right side (A), rotating the leg outward as much as possible for a few reps and then inward as much as possible for a few reps. This rotation is critical to the effectiveness of this movement. Next, swing your right leg across to the left in front of your body (B), again rotating the leg outward for a few reps and then inward for a few reps. Next, swing your right leg out to your right side once again (C), again rotating it outward for a few reps then inward for a few reps. Then swing the leg across to the left behind your body (D), once again rotating it outward for a few reps then inward for a few reps. Repeat on the other side. Work up to as many pain-free reps as you can before switching to the other side.

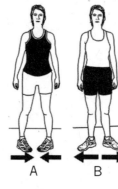

Standing Toes In and Out

Piriformis, iliopsoas, hamstrings, gluteus medius, gluteus minimus, gluteus maximus, soleus

Stand for a time with your toes pointed inward (A), then stand with your toes pointed outward (B). Gradually adopting a more extreme inward and outward position over time may seem like a very slight movement, but it's very beneficial for the psoas, the hamstrings, and, especially, the gluteal muscles.

Other exercises that will benefit the piriformis

- Hamstrings protocol
  - Walking uphill with toes in and out

Range of Motion Protocol for Hamstrings

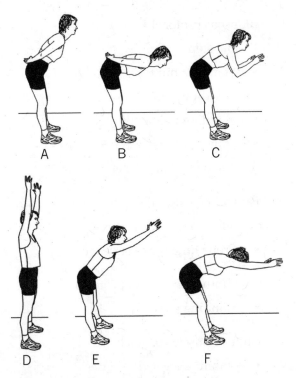

A   B   C

D   E   F

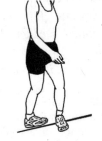

Walking Uphill with Toes In and Out

Hamstrings, soleus, gluteus medius, gluteus minimus, gluteus maximus, piriformis

Walking uphill with your toes pointing in for a while and then pointing out for a while is an almost effortless way to increase range of motion for the hamstrings, gluteal muscles, and soleus. For greater benefit, just walk a longer distance or up a steeper incline, but don't do more than you can without pain.

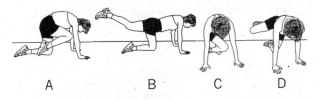

A   B   C   D

All-Fours Series

Hamstrings, iliopsoas, gluteus maximus, gluteus medius, gluteus minimus, piriformis

From an all-fours position, bring your right knee to your chest (A), then swing your right leg back and up (B). Swing your right knee forward again, but this time across your chest toward your left elbow (C). Bring your right leg out to the side and up to about hip level, keeping the knee bent (D). Bring your right leg back down to the starting position. At first, alternate legs with each repetition. As you gain strength and flexibility, do multiple reps with each leg before switching to the other leg.

Forward Torso Bend Series

Hamstrings, paraspinals, gluteus maximus, rectus abdominis, soleus

Beginner: Stand upright with your knees straight and your hands behind your back. Slowly bend forward at your hips with your back straight (A), bending as far as you can without pain. Slowly return to the starting position. Over time, bend farther until you can achieve a 90-degree forward bend (B).

Intermediate: Stand with your arms up, elbows bent, with your hands in front of your face. Slowly bend forward at your hips with your back straight, bending as far as you can without pain (C). Slowly return to the starting position. Over time, bend farther until you can achieve a 90-degree forward bend.

Advanced: Start with both arms extended overhead (D). Slowly bend forward at your hips with your back straight (E). Bend as far as you can without pain, keeping your arms at the level of your ears. Slowly return to the starting position. Over time, work up to a full 90-degree forward bend (F).

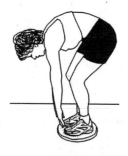

Dynamic Standing and Bending

Hamstrings, rectus abdominis, paraspinals, gluteus maximus, gluteus medius, gluteus minimus, quadratus lumborum, soleus, iliopsoas

Stand balanced on both feet on a surface that will be wobbly when you stand on it, like a dynamic seating disk partially filled with air, a balance or wobble board, a piece of dense foam, or a pillow. Exhale and slowly bend forward, slightly bending your knees and keeping your balance as you touch your toes or the floor with your fingertips, keeping your abdominal muscles relaxed. Inhale and slowly straighten your back to return to a standing position. This movement requires good balance. Until you've mastered it, lightly grasp a sturdy chair or other support to help you keep your balance.

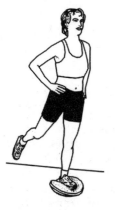

Dynamic Standing on One Leg

Hamstrings, gluteus maximus, soleus, paraspinals, iliopsoas

Beginner: It's best to work up to this standing on one leg on a dynamic surface by first practicing standing on one leg on a regular floor. Once you can do that for one minute, move up to the intermediate level.

Intermediate: Stand balanced on one foot on a surface that will be wobbly when you stand on it, like a dynamic seating disk partially filled with air, a balance or wobble board, a piece of dense foam, or a pillow. Start by trying to balance for 10 seconds, and increase the length of time as you progress. Until you've really mastered this movement, lightly grasp a sturdy chair or table to help maintain your balance. Repeat on the other side.

Advanced: While standing and balancing on one foot on the dynamic surface, slowly bend down toward the floor, then return to an upright position. If you're really good at this, you can try picking up a light weight from the floor.

Other exercises that will benefit the hamstrings

- Iliopsoas protocol
  - Big steps
  - Standing hip twist
  - Standing toes in and out
  - Standing pelvic tilt
  - Standing twist and bend series
  - Torso bend and extend series

- Paraspinals protocol
  - Superman
  - Prone fitness ball series

- Quadratus lumborum protocol
  - Standing twist

- Gluteal muscles protocol
  - Standing leg swing series
  - Grapevine series

- Soleus protocol
  - Walking uphill
  - Knee bend series

Range of Motion Protocol for Soleus

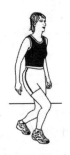

Walking with Knees Bent

Soleus

It's easy to increase range of motion exercise for the soleus by incorporating variations in the way you walk as you go about your day. For example, while walking, bend your knees after you've stepped forward. Keep your heels on the floor, then take another step forward.

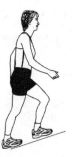

Walking Uphill

Soleus, hamstrings, gluteus maximus, gluteus medius, gluteus minimus, iliopsoas

Walking uphill is a great way to stretch and exercise the soleus and increase range of motion for other muscles.

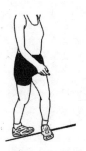

Walking Uphill with Toes In and Out

Soleus, gluteus medius, gluteus maximus, gluteus minimus, hamstrings, piriformis

For more variation and increased range of motion, walk uphill with your toes pointing in for a while and then pointing out for a while.

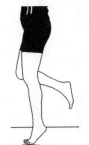

Single Heel Raise

Soleus

Balance on your left foot, then slowly raise yourself up onto the ball of your foot, rising as high as you can without pain. Slowly lower your heel to the ground. If necessary, lightly grasp a sturdy chair or table for balance. Work up to as many pain-free reps as you can before switching to the other side.

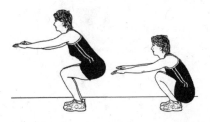

Knee Bend Series

Soleus, gluteus maximus, paraspinals, hamstrings

Beginner: When you first start doing this exercise, stand in a doorway where you can hold on to the doorjamb for balance and assistance in returning to a standing position. Grasp the doorjamb at about waist level, then bend your knees and slowly bring your buttocks toward the floor, going as far as you can while keeping your heels on the floor. Slowly return to a standing position.

Intermediate: Once you no longer need the doorjamb for balance and support, do the exercise exactly as in the beginner version, but without holding onto a support.

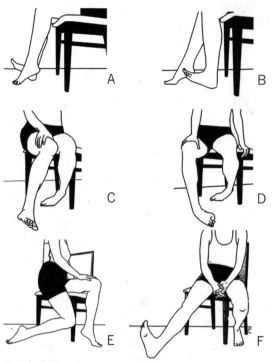

Pedal Series

Soleus

While seated, point your left foot down and flex your right foot up (A). Switch and point your right foot down and flex your left foot up (B). Next, pull your left foot back, out of the way, and roll your right foot inward (C), then outward (D). Next, relax your calf and place the top of your right foot on the floor behind you (E), twisting in the chair if need be. Then extend your right leg in front of you, straightening the knee and flexing your right ankle (F). Repeat the entire sequence on the other side. It's a good idea to do this series frequently throughout the day.

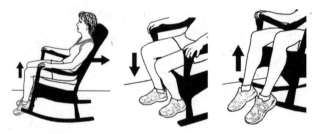

Rocking Chair

Soleus

The natural motion involved in rocking in a chair is very therapeutic for the soleus. Push off the floor with your toes, and be sure to allow your heels to return fully to the floor before pressing back up. Continue rocking for at least 10 minutes—or much longer if you like!

Other exercises that will benefit the soleus

- Iliopsoas protocol
  - Big steps
  - Standing hip twist
  - Standing toes in and out
  - Seated flex and extension
  - Torso bend and extend series
  - Standing pelvic tilt
  - Standing twist and bend series

- Rectus abdominis protocol
  - Dynamic standing and bending

- Quadratus lumborum protocol
  - Standing hip swing
  - Standing hip hike
  - Standing twist
  - Standing side stretch
  - Standing side bend

- Gluteal muscles protocol
  - Standing leg swing series
  - Grapevine series

- Hamstrings protocol
  - Forward torso bend series
  - Dynamic standing and bending
  - Dynamic standing on one leg

Chapter 17

General Perpetuating Factors

We've described how trigger points and referred pain cause many different kinds of low back and buttocks pain, and we've also listed many factors that may cause trigger point activation for each muscle or muscle group covered in this book. Those causes can generally be divided into two categories: precipitating or aggravating factors (specific incidents, actions, or situations that initiate pain) and perpetuating factors (those that can not only cause pain, but also keep a pain problem going and sometimes make it worse, despite effective trigger point therapy). A precipitating factor could be lifting a heavy object without bending your knees. A perpetuating factor could be working at a desk in an ergonomically poor seated position.

If your pain began recently and was caused by an accident, trauma, or stressful situation or action, self-care treatment will usually relieve the pain and fix the problem. But if you've been living with pain for some time, unrecognized perpetuating factors may be sustaining the problem, even if you do get temporary relief from self-care treatment. In such cases, to resolve the problem fully you need to consider what's perpetuating or exacerbating the trigger points. In this chapter, we'll review perpetuating factors in general and cover some of the more common perpetuating factors for low back and buttocks pain more extensively. It's worth your while to read this chapter closely, as these perpetuating factors are often overlooked by health care professionals.

Drs. Travell and Simons broadly classified the causes of trigger points into the following categories:

- Traumatic injuries, such as slips or falls

- Chemical imbalances

- Nutritional factors

- Psychological factors

- Mechanical factors

Traumatic injuries are precipitating factors; the other categories are usually considered to be perpetuating factors. We'll discuss mechanical factors more extensively below, but first let's consider the other three types of perpetuating factors to see how they may be contributing to your pain.

Chemical Imbalances and Nutritional Factors

In our view, nutritional factors are closely related to chemical imbalances, so we'll discuss those two categories together.

Chemical Imbalances

Chemical imbalances, such as hormone imbalances (including thyroid) and vitamin and mineral deficiencies and insufficiencies, are often an important contributing factor. Thyroid hormone imbalance can sometimes be a problem even when standard tests indicate a person is within the normal range. So even if your tests indicate normal levels or your doctor says that your levels are normal, if you have common symptoms of low thyroid function such as systemic pain, chronic fatigue, muscle cramping, hair loss, or cold extremities, you might consider working with a specialist who is willing to do further testing or treat you based on your symptoms.

Nutritional Factors

For our purposes, nutrition is a broad category that extends beyond food to encompass all of the substances you ingest. Here are some of the more common nutritional problems that can cause or exacerbate muscle pain. If any of these factors apply to you and your pain persists despite effective self-care treatment, you may need to address them directly to achieve lasting pain relief:

- Insufficient vitamins or minerals in the diet

- Lack of sufficient hydration, which is often exacerbated by diuretics used to reduce weight or blood pressure

- Irregular eating habits, including bingeing or going without food for extended periods

- Smoking or excessive alcohol consumption, which can cause or exacerbate dehydration and depletion of nutrients

- Prescription medications with side effects that can cause or exacerbate chronic muscle pain and dysfunction

Whenever you attempt to address a long-standing condition or a habit like smoking or irregular eating patterns, simple awareness seldom suffices to correct the problem. We don't claim special expertise in treating or changing such habits and conditions, but there are many books, programs, and other resources that can help. In general, you'll need to come up with a specific plan for changing and commit to following it. Most experts believe that it takes at least three to four weeks to change a habit, so don't expect overnight success. You may find it helpful to replace the habit with a new behavior, such as the self-care techniques, stretches, and range of motion exercises in this book. Also, don't underestimate the importance of support from others in changing your habits.

With some nutritional problems, you may need to consult a physician or specialist to determine the exact nature of the problem, its possible effects on chronic pain, and how to treat it. For other nutritional factors, you can conduct simple experiments to see if changing your behavior for a limited time changes your pain. One fairly common problem that's simple to correct is insufficient hydration. If you think this may be a factor for you, try increasing your water intake to a minimum of 8 cups daily, in addition to other fluids, and see if this reduces your pain. If this is a perpetuating factor for you, you should see a noticeable reduction in pain.

Overreliance on prescription medications for pain is a serious problem. Trigger points aren't eliminated by medication; medication simply masks the pain they cause and only does so for short periods. And over time, many people require more medication to achieve the same level of relief. In many cases, the side effects of medication can actually exacerbate myofascial pain. If you have trigger points and myofascial pain, long-term use of painkillers isn't in your best interests. You should work with your physician to wean yourself from these medications as you continue to do your self-care treatment.

Vitamin or Mineral Deficiencies and Insufficiencies

Vitamin or mineral *deficiency* technically refers to abnormally low levels of nutrients. The term *insufficiency* refers to levels at the low end of the normal range. Deficiencies, as well as insufficiencies, can create a predisposition to activation of trigger points and perpetuation of myofascial pain syndromes. One study of chronic pain patients determined that 89 percent of those tested had insufficient blood levels of vitamin D, with only 28 percent having levels low enough to be considered deficient (Plotnikoff and Quigley 2003). So, clinically "normal" levels of vitamin D are still capable of contributing to chronic pain.

If you find that self-care treatment doesn't provide lasting pain relief and you've considered and ruled out the other perpetuating factors in this chapter, it would be worthwhile to have testing to determine whether insufficiency of one or more nutrients may be a perpetuating factor for you. Be aware that even if you test within the normal range, you may have vitamin or mineral insufficiencies that could account for the persistence of myofascial pain after regular trigger point treatment. To help you interpret your test results, see the table below, which is based on research conducted by neurologist and pain expert Robert Gerwin (2005), as well as personal communication with and clinical evidence compiled by Dr. Anna Bittner and Dr. Tim Taylor, experts in the field of myofascial pain. If you test below the lower end of any range or level in the table, insufficiency of that vitamin or mineral could be a significant perpetuating factor in your pain. (Also note that excessive levels of the fat-soluble vitamins A, D, and E can also perpetuate chronic myofascial pain, but this is highly unlikely.)

For TSH (thyroid stimulating hormone), values above 2.5 warrant further investigation for possible hypothyroidism (Gerwin 2005). Note also that serum level of ferritin is preferred over general iron levels because serum ferritin best indicates the body's store of iron available for muscle. Ferritin levels below 50ng/ml have been associated with restless leg syndrome symptoms. (Wang et al 2009; Bittner and Taylor 2009).

Useful Lab Tests		
	Men	**Women**
	Your clinical test results should be at or greater than these values	
Ferritin (a storage form of iron)	50 ng/ml	50 ng/ml
Vitamin B$_1$ (thiamin)	4.0 mcg/l	4.0 mcg/l
Vitamin B$_6$	5.4–6.7 mcg/l	2.0–2.8 mcg/l
Vitamin B$_{12}$	350 pg/ml	350 pg/ml
Vitamin D	50 ng/ml	50 ng/ml
Serum folate	5.4 mg/ml	5.4 mg/ml
	Your clinical test results should be within these ranges	
Serum calcium	8.5–10.6 mg/dl	8.5–10.6 mg/dl
Vitamin C	0.4–2.0 mg/dl	0.4–2.0 mg/dl
TSH	0.4–2.0 microIU/ml	0.4–2.0 microIU/ml
Serum magnesium	1.8–3.0 mg/dl	1.8–3.0 mg/dl
Serum potassium	3.5–5.2 mmol/l	3.5–5.2 mmol/l

If you decide to get tested for vitamin and mineral insufficiencies, be sure to insist on testing for vitamin D, which is often overlooked. Some practitioners don't even know the name for the test: 25 hydroxy-vitamin D serum test. Keep in mind that sunlight is an important source of vitamin D, and because so many people have been warned to avoid direct sunlight, an increasing percentage of the population may be susceptible to vitamin D insufficiency. Low levels of vitamin D require aggressive supplementation, and even with that, the deficiency could take as long as three months to correct (Gerwin 2005; Taylor and Bittner 2009; Wang et al. 2009). According to Dr. Tim Taylor and Dr. Anna Bittner of Pain Relief Home in Richmond, Virginia, "For vitamin D insufficiency, we use the fastest dosage that has been published as safe and effective: Vitamin D3 50,000 IU prescription one per day with a fat-containing meal for one month, then one per week for a month, then retest. We are getting complete vitamin D recovery to desirable ranges in almost all of our patients within the two-month period."

If testing indicates that you have vitamin or mineral insufficiencies, it's best to consult a physician or licensed dietitian to determine the best way to correct the imbalance, as it can be more complicated than simply taking a multivitamin daily. Because more detailed recommendations are beyond the scope of this book, we primarily want to emphasize that you can't simply rely on the currently used parameters of vitamin and mineral deficiencies. Each person's "normal" value can be different.

Psychological Factors

The range of psychological factors that can contribute to pain is vast; a thorough discussion is beyond our expertise and beyond the purview of this book. What we can say is that we have observed patients with high levels of anxiety that resulted in myofascial trigger points, pain, and dysfunction, including poor posture, overall muscle tension, or disordered breathing. If anxiety is an issue, it could result in specific problems such as paradoxical breathing, shallow breathing, overbreathing, or an unconscious habit of holding the body in a state of perpetual tension. While we can't treat the underlying anxiety, we can hardly avoid noticing its physical manifestations. In such cases, we try to help the patient become more conscious of the muscle tension the anxiety is causing. We also help patients retrain the muscles to relax through self-care treatment, stretching, and exercise. Do note that it can take up to four months of steady retraining to overcome long-standing breathing disorders and habitual muscle tension.

If your goal is lasting pain relief, try to assess whether anxiety affects your breathing patterns and general state of muscle tension. If you suspect that anxiety is a significant factor, don't just continue to live with it. Seek help from a qualified therapist who can help you overcome your anxiety and the physical habits associated with it. Self-treatment using the techniques in this book will also help by making you aware of your muscle tension and thereby serving as a type of biofeedback process. If the underlying perpetuating factor is muscle tension from anxiety, you can learn to stop holding this tension in your muscles.

One specific form of disordered breathing is particularly problematic. Known as *paradoxical breathing*, it involves tightening the neck muscles, chest, and abdomen when you inhale—the opposite of a normal, healthy breathing pattern. This leads to overuse of the upper chest and neck muscles. Although paradoxical breathing may be caused by purely physical factors, it can also arise for psychological reasons. The same is true of other abnormal breathing patterns, so all are worth investigating, no matter what their cause. Here are some of the common symptoms of abnormal breathing:

- Tightening the neck when inhaling

- Tightening the abdomen when inhaling

- Holding the abdomen in to look more fit

- Pain and dysfunction in any part of the upper body

- Holding one's breath (often unconsciously)

- Dizziness or light-headedness

- Tingling in the hands during or after slight exertion

- Frequent feelings of anxiety

- An inability to take deep breaths

- Frequent yawning or sighing

- Mouth breathing or a dry mouth

- Difficulty concentrating

- Feeling out of breath after mild exertion

- Pain and dysfunction in the neck, arms, head, and chest activated by exercise

If you experience any of these symptoms, your breathing patterns may be playing a role in perpetuating your pain. Fortunately, simple exercises can often help correct disordered breathing if practiced over time. Here's one we recommend. As you do this exercise, focus on breathing in a way that helps you feel calm and relaxed, rather than on breathing deeply:

1. Lie down on your back with your knees bent.

2. Place your left hand over your belly and your right hand at the side of your neck, pressing in lightly.

3. Relax your abdomen and allow your belly (and hand) to rise as you slowly inhale, breathing through your nose with your tongue pressed against the roof of your mouth.

4. Use your right hand to feel whether your neck muscles tighten as you inhale. If they do, try to breathe in such a way that they don't.

5. Next, focus on your breathing as you exhale slowly and without strain. As you exhale, your left hand should go down.

If you determine that your breathing pattern is a problem, incorporate this exercise as part of your daily self-care routine for at least 5 minutes a day for the first week. Then gradually increase to 10 and then 15 minutes daily. As you learn this natural breathing style, do it in a semirecumbent position, then practice it while sitting, and after a few weeks, practice it while standing. Finally, practice breathing in this way while you're walking and performing daily activities. Changing your breathing pattern may take time, though some people can learn fairly quickly. Remember, you aren't trying to breathe deeply; you're trying to breathe in a way that helps you remain calm and relaxed.

Some people tighten their muscles in response to any direction to change their breathing pattern. If you feel fear, increased anxiety, dizziness, or increased pain as you do this breathing exercise, you aren't doing it correctly. If this happens, realize that this is quite common and try to find a way to relax. If the problem persists, you need to take it more slowly or discontinue the work on breathing, at least temporarily. You might seek professional help to get started on breathing exercises and improving your breathing pattern. If that sounds silly, remember that breathing is the most elemental function of life, so any improvement you can make is extremely valuable. Because breathing is so fundamental, it can be a central part of the problem, as well as the easiest perpetuating factor to overlook. If you need further information about breathing pattern disorders, their consequences, and appropriate methods of treatment, we recommend the book *Multidisciplinary Approaches to Breathing Pattern Disorders* (Chaitow, Bradley, and Gilbert 2002).

Mechanical Factors

Nobody's perfect. This idea is easy to embrace as a generality. But how often do you consider this in relation to your own body? Each of us has some body part that's slightly bigger, longer, fuller, or just plain different. Slight physical asymmetries usually don't cause problems, but beyond a certain point they can activate trigger points, and this can occur on either the side that's shorter or the side that's longer. There are several common structural asymmetries or imbalances that often play a role in low back and buttocks pain, and in our clinical experience, many people who suffer from chronic pain are affected by one or more of them. In addition, muscular problems can cause or exacerbate structural asymmetries. It's important to consider these factors and deal with them if they're present.

Before we get into the details, we want to make two overarching points: First, it's astonishing how frequently we see very noticeable structural imbalances that have never been detected or reported in a prior physical examination. And second, it's also amazing how often a simple, inexpensive correction to such an imbalance will bring about a significant reduction in pain. In the majority of cases, correcting the imbalance combined with self-care treatment is the key to lasting pain relief. We cannot overstress how important it is to detect structural imbalances and correct them. With that introduction, let's take a closer look at some of the structural imbalances and mechanical factors that most commonly result in myofascial dysfunction:

- Small hemipelvis

- Leg length inequality

- Morton's foot syndrome

- Poor footwear choices

- Short upper arms

- Problems related to sleep position

Small Hemipelvis

If you're sitting while reading this book, reach under your buttocks and feel your sit bones, also known as the ischial tuberosities. These bones are located at the bottom of the pelvic structure and bear most of your weight when you sit. When one side of the pelvis is smaller than the other, the smaller side is referred to as a small hemipelvis. In figure 17.1A, the right side is smaller. If you have a small hemipelvis, it will make you uneven whenever you sit, which can cause trigger points to develop throughout much of the body—in the head, neck, shoulders, hips, buttocks, legs, and upper, mid, and lower

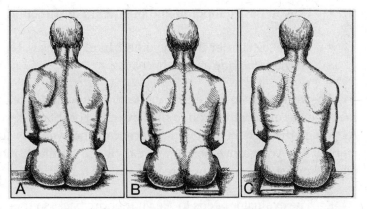

Figure 17.1

back. Such trigger points are one of the most common causes of sciatica and pain in the low back, buttocks, hips, and legs. An uneven pelvis can also lead to scoliosis, a condition in which the spine is curved to the side, as you can also see in figure 17.1A.

In general, a small hemipelvis means you'll be sitting slightly slanted to one side. This chronic tilt sends signals to the brain that activate the righting reflex. In response, your head might tilt to the opposite side to maintain a level position. This can set off a chain of muscular interactions that leave some muscles in a chronic state of overuse, which in turn leads to myofascial pain and dysfunction. Another common response to this structural imbalance is to try to correct the pelvic tilt by crossing one leg over the other.

Testing for a Small Hemipelvis

To determine whether you may have a small hemipelvis, ask yourself the following questions:

- Do you often sit with one foot tucked under your buttocks?

- Do you have a hard time sitting for long periods?

- Do you have a hard time finding a comfortable seated position?

- When sitting, do you usually cross one leg over the other if you can?

- Do you have back pain when sitting?

- Do you avoid sitting?

- Do you prefer to work in a standing position?

- Do you have headaches?

- Do you have temporomandibular joint dysfunction (TMJD)?

- Is one leg shorter than the other? In many cases, the vertical height of the pelvis is smaller on the same side as the short leg.

Answering yes to any of these questions may indicate that you have a small hemipelvis, in which case you should continue on to the next test. For this test, you'll need another person to evaluate you. As you go through the following procedure, the evaluator (the other person) should record any asymmetries. For your convenience, we've included an illustration of the back of the body, which you can photocopy for the evaluator to record any asymmetries.

1. The evaluator needs to see your entire back, so if possible you should remove all clothing from your upper body.

2. Sit on a level, hard seat without a backrest, such as a wooden piano bench. Alternatively, you can sit on a hard board on a stool or a softer chair without a backrest.

3. The evaluator should first look at the base of your skull and your ears. Is your head tilted? It helps to use a yardstick or even a carpenter's level to measure whether one ear is higher

Postural Assessment Sheet

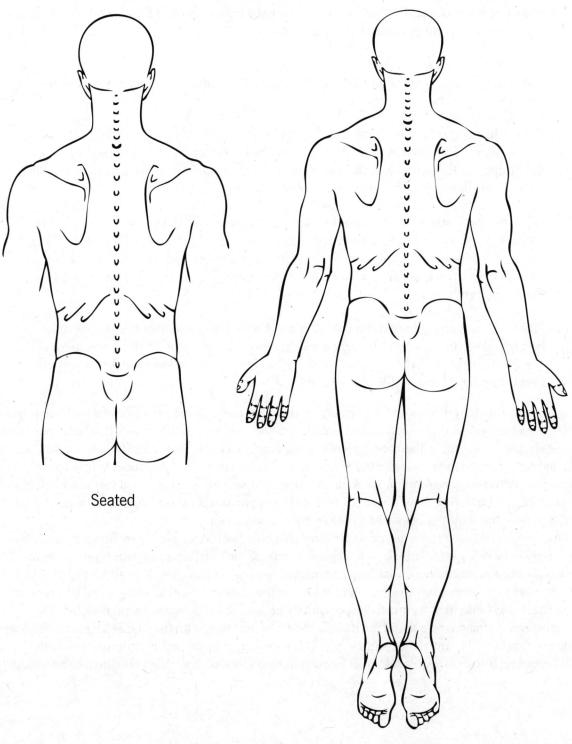

Seated

Standing

Use this sheet to record your findings.

or lower than the other. On the assessment sheet, draw a line to indicate the finding, making it horizontal if the ears are level, or slightly tilted if they're uneven.

4. Next the evaluator should measure the top of your shoulder blades, noticing if one is higher or if one of the shoulder blades seems to bulge outward. Again, draw a line on the assessment sheet to indicate the finding.

5. Next the evaluator should feel for the bottom tips of your shoulder blades and measure to determine whether one is higher than the other. Mark any difference on the assessment sheet.

6. The evaluator should then press their hands into the sides of your waist and feel the iliac crest to determine whether one side is higher. The evaluator should also measure whether the dimples of the pelvis near the top of the sacrum are higher on one side than the other. Indicate the findings on the assessment sheet.

7. From the back, the evaluator should then observe the way the spine lines up from the sacrum. Are the vertebrae stacked up straight, or do they curve from side to side? It can be easier to see the shape of the spine if the spinous process of each vertebra is marked with a pen. This makes it easier to see any abnormal curvature. Again, indicate the finding on the assessment sheet.

8. Finally, look at any skin folds on the sides and back of the torso. Are they larger or deeper on one side than the other? If there are differences, draw them on the assessment sheet. The evaluator should also observe whether these folds tend to even out when you place a butt lift under the small side of the pelvis.

If this examination reveals any asymmetries, this may indicate the presence of a small hemipelvis. In that case, the next step is to correct the imbalance and notice any differences that you feel. You can make a simple ischial lift using the pages of a magazine. Place the lift under the shorter side, starting with enough pages to measure about 1/8 inch. Does this correct the imbalance? If this feels good but insufficient, add more pages, about 1/8 inch at a time, and keep assessing how it feels and how it looks. In figure 17.1B, above, note how the small hemipelvis is corrected by putting a lift under the right sit bone, and how the shoulder blades and iliac crests are now even.

Once you've achieved symmetry, to confirm that this is an effective correction for you, place the magazine on the other side. This should accentuate any pelvic imbalance, as you can see in figure 17.1C, above, making you more uncomfortable. You might even feel as though you're about to fall over, and it may increase your pain. Have your evaluator look at the same physical landmarks as before. With the lift on the second side, any asymmetries previously noted should be more pronounced.

Now take the magazine out and put it back under the first side, with the suspected small hemipelvis. If you've corrected the imbalance sufficiently, you should feel a noticeable difference in both comfort and symmetry. If so, you've just taken an important step toward changing your life for the better!

Correcting for a Small Hemipelvis

Now sit on the magazine for 5 to 10 minutes. Ask your evaluator to check the same physical landmarks as before:

- Has your head leveled out? Are your ears more even?

- Are your shoulders even?

- Are your shoulder blades even?

- How about the bones of the iliac crest, just below the waist?

- How about any skin folds?

- Has your overall pain abated somewhat?

Next, take the magazine out and measure the thickness. This is the thickness you'll need for your butt lift. If these tests indicate you have a small hemipelvis, be sure that your self-care routine devotes special attention to all of the muscles on either side that have been chronically shortened or lengthened, especially the quadratus lumborum, spinal erectors, abdominals, and gluteal muscles.

You'll also need to find or make a lift to give extra height to the sit bone on the short side. This can be as simple as a small magazine, a notepad, or even a folded washcloth. You need to use this correction whenever you sit: at work, at home, in the car, at a place of worship, at the movies, and so on. On softer surfaces, you'll need a higher lift (as much as double) because the sit bones and the buttocks as a whole will tend to sink into the surface.

If you don't consult a health care professional and obtain X-rays to confirm the pelvic inequality, it's important to continue monitoring your seated position and reaction to it over time. Keep in mind that myofascial dysfunction can cause a false positive, meaning the tests may indicate that you have a small hemipelvis, but extensive self-care, including compression and stretching of the affected muscles, may correct and equalize the muscular imbalance that caused it. If the imbalance that caused the asymmetry was more muscular than skeletal, it may eventually be possible to use a shorter lift or even phase it out altogether.

Of course, you can take a more rigorous approach to this entire process and enlist the aid of a physiatrist, chiropractor, MD, or osteopath, who can order seated X-rays and measure the pelvis from the iliac crest to the ischial tuberosity. That said, with due diligence most people are capable of performing the testing and correction described here without consulting a professional. In either case, the key is using precise measurements to ensure the ischial lift corrects the asymmetry properly.

Leg Length Inequality

While the actual length of the leg bones can vary, muscular dysfunction and other physical issues can also affect leg length, including how the spine and sacrum interact with the pelvis and how the feet and ankles align when bearing weight. If the inequality is caused by muscles that contain trigger points, they can be easily treated and corrected. Whatever the cause or extent of leg length inequality, a variety of muscles may act to counter this condition and develop trigger points as a result of both underuse and

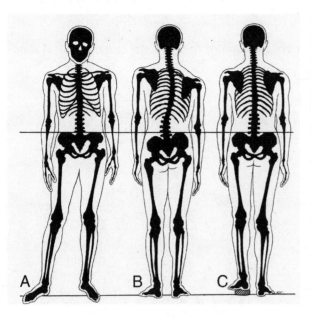

Figure 17.2

overuse, particularly the quadratus lumborum, the paraspinals, the iliopsoas, the abdominals, and all the gluteal muscles. We find this condition to be fairly common, and generally uncorrected, so it makes sense to check for leg length inequality. There are many possible responses to leg length inequality, as you can see in figure 17.2. In figure 17.2A, a front view, the spine stays straight but the person has shifted their weight to the left leg, allowing the longer right let to extend off to the side. In figure 17.2B, a back view, both legs bear an equal amount of weight; because the right leg is longer, the pelvis tilts, the spine curves, and the shoulders and hips are uneven.

In figure 17.2C, a heel lift has been placed under the short left leg to correct the inequality. This in turn will help to level the pelvis, normalize the spinal curves and level the shoulders and head. It should also be noted that a dysfunctional SI (sacroiliac) joint can also cause a pseudo-leg length inequality as it can cause one to stand with the leg turned out, pelvic rotation and pain when standing. (Simons 2009) Since this leg length has probably been uncorrected for a long time, all dysfunctional muscles noted on the bottom of page 241 will need trigger point therapy.

Testing for Standing Leg Length Inequality

Unless you have X-rays to measure the bones, you'll have to check for the characteristic anomalies that occur with leg length inequality. Ask yourself the following questions:

- Do you tend to stand mostly on one leg?

- Do you typically stand on one leg with the other leg forward and to the side, sometimes accompanied by a hand on the hip?

- Does your back pain increase when you stand?

- Is your back pain mostly on one side?

- Does your pelvis tend to have a very limited range of movement either forward and backward or from side to side?

Answering yes to any of these questions may indicate leg length inequality, in which case you should do the next test, which is similar to testing for a small hemipelvis except that it's conducted in a standing position. You'll need another person to evaluate you. As you go through the following procedures, the evaluator should record any asymmetries on the illustration of the back of the body found earlier in this chapter.

1. It's best to be able to observe the entire back, so if possible remove all clothing from your upper body.

2. Stand facing away from the evaluator with your feet shoulder width apart. Make sure the floor in the room is level.

3. The evaluator should first look at the back of the skull and the level of the ears. Are they even? Again, it helps to use a yardstick or a carpenter's level to measure whether the ears are level.

4. The evaluator should measure the top of your shoulder blades to determine whether one is higher or one seems to bulge outward.

5. Next, the evaluator should feel for the bottom tips of your shoulder blades and measure whether one is higher. If the leg length inequality is 1/2 inch or more, the shoulder is usually lower on the side of the shorter leg.

6. Next, the evaluator should press their hands into the sides of your waist and feel for the iliac crest of the hip. Is one side higher than the other side?

7. The evaluator should then measure whether the dimples of the pelvis near the top of the sacrum are higher on one side than the other.

8. Then the evaluator should stand behind and observe the way the spine stacks up from the sacrum. Is the spine straight or does it curve to the right or left? To facilitate this evaluation, small pen marks can be made on the spinous process of each vertebra, and then these marks can be connected with a line. If there is a noticeable curvature, take a picture of it and use it as a baseline for comparison after you've completed at least four weeks of self-care treatment.

9. Finally, the evaluator should look at any skin folds on the sides and back of the torso. Are they deeper on one side than the other? When you correct for the short leg, you should notice the skin folds evening out.

Correcting for Standing Leg Length Inequality

Based on this assessment, you should be able to determine whether you have standing leg length inequality due to either differences in bone length or muscular dysfunction. If you do, the next step is to make corrections gradually and carefully note any changes in the asymmetries that were observed in the assessment.

Start by placing a magazine approximately 1/8 inch thick under the foot of the leg that seems shorter. Does this help even out any asymmetries? If the lift makes your back more level but it's still uneven, add more height to the lift until your shoulders, hips, and any skin folds appear completely even, as in figure 17.2C. Bear in mind that for this to be a good correction, it has to feel noticeably more comfortable. You should feel more level, balanced, and strong. To confirm that you've made the appropriate correction, transfer the lift underneath the foot of the other leg (the "long" leg). If leg length inequality is an issue for you, you'll immediately feel more uneven, unstable, and uncomfortable at the hips and shoulders. Once you've confirmed this condition, you can acquire heel lifts with the same amount of correction to place in your shoe on the short side.

Quite often, people with leg length inequality feel an almost immediate reduction in pain once the problem is corrected with a heel lift. However, all of the muscles affected by the leg length inequality still require treatment, including the quadratus lumborum, paraspinals, abdominals, psoas, hamstrings, and soleus. Comprehensive self-care treatment of all of these muscles will help ensure that they return to full pain-free function. You may need to do self-care up to four times daily at first. As with a small hemipelvis, it's important to reevaluate after a while to see if you need to continue using the heel lift on a long-term basis. After you've treated and retrained the muscles sufficiently, you may be able to gradually reduce the size of the lift or even eliminate it completely.

Morton's Foot Syndrome

In the 1940s, Dr. Dudley J. Morton discovered significant variations in the shape of foot bones among a standard patient population. If your second toe appears to be the longest of your toes or if the space between your first and second toe cuts deeper into the foot than does the space between your second and third toe, you may have Morton's foot syndrome. Other indications include bunions or calluses on the ball of the foot, especially behind the second toe. Although the incidence of this condition isn't that high in the general population, among people with chronic myofascial pain the incidence is very high. People with Morton's foot syndrome also have an elevated and *supinated* first metatarsal, meaning it's elevated and rotated outward. (The metatarsals are the bones that extend from the toes into the ball of the foot.)

With this condition, the big toe (which normally carries most of your weight) is elevated so it carries hardly any weight. For it to reach the ground, the arch must drop and the ankle must roll in. This leads to the condition known as *hyperpronation*, in which the inside edge of the foot falls inward. People with this condition often walk duck-footed, with their feet splayed outward. Hyperpronation changes how the ankle moves, how the knee travels over the foot, how the thigh bone sits in the hip socket, how the gluteal muscles act on the hip, how the spine is aligned, how the head sits on the spine, and how the jaw, or temporomandibular joint, functions. All of these imbalances can lead to muscular overload, trigger points, nerve compression, sciatica, piriformis syndrome, and other forms of chronic pain. So even though hyperpronation is a foot and ankle condition, it's often associated with knee, hip, low back, buttocks, upper back, neck, head, and jaw pain.

Testing for Morton's Foot Syndrome

It's pretty simple to determine whether or not you have Morton's foot syndrome. Just sit down, take your shoes and socks off, and take a look.

- Is the space between your first and second toes deeper than the space between your second and third toes?

- Does it look like your second toe is longer than your big toe? (Note that this isn't always the case, and that the depth of the space between the toes is the major determinant.) If you have sufficient knowledge of anatomy, you can also look to see if the second metatarsal bone seems longer.

- Look at your old shoes. Are the wear patterns uneven? Are they worn more on the outside or inside of the heel? Are they worn at the ball of the foot between the first and second toes? Uneven shoe wear, like uneven tire wear, usually means trouble.

- Look at the bottom of your feet. Do you have calluses on the outside edge of your big toe, in the middle of the ball of the foot, or on the ball of the foot between the second and third toe? Do you have calluses on the back or inside edge of your heel? Such calluses are a classic symptom of Morton's foot syndrome and can be painful.

- Do you have a bunion? Does your big toe lie at an angle, pushing the other toes over toward the outside of your foot?

- Do you tend to stand or walk with your feet rotated outward, like a duck? Does it feel like your ankles are rolling or falling inward, or do your feet feel unstable and your ankles weak?

- When walking alongside people, do you often bump into the person walking to your left or right?

If you answer yes to any of these questions, you probably have Morton's foot syndrome. If so, when you walk, most of your weight is distributed between your heel and the second toe bone, almost as if you were walking on ice skates. If this causes your ankles and feet to collapse inward, or hyperpronate, this may well be a major cause of neck, shoulder, ankle, knee, hip, or back pain. It's also likely that you've always had generally poor posture. Another possibility is that you brace or tighten your leg muscles all the way up to the hip to prevent the ankle from collapsing inward. In either case, if you have Morton's foot syndrome, your feet aren't working right. You spend too much time on either the inside or outside of your feet and too little time in a balanced, stable position with good body mechanics and relaxed muscles.

Fortunately, dealing with an elevated first metatarsal is simple and inexpensive. You need only place a wedge (described more fully below) beneath your first metatarsal. This will ensure that your big toe meets the ground sooner in the weight-bearing cycle.

Correcting for Morton's Foot Syndrome

The next step is to determine how much you need to build up underneath the first metatarsal and big toe in order to prevent your ankles from collapsing. To measure this, you can use a small pad of Post-it notes; this is ideal because you can adjust the height by very small increments. Start with enough Post-it notes to elevate your toe about 6 to 7 millimeters (about 1/4 inch). Don't let the Post-it notes infringe on the second toe or your arch. Do a few knee bends, leaning slightly forward and keeping your heels on the ground. Are your ankles stable now? If they still roll inward or your knees still track inward, place more Post-it notes under the big toe until you stabilize the arch and ankle.

When you have enough Post-it notes to provide stability, measure the stack of them using a metric ruler. If the stack measures 7 millimeters or less, you'll benefit from a 3.5-millimeter lift underneath the first metatarsal and big toe. If the amount needed to bring your ankle and lower leg bone into alignment is more than 7 millimeters, you'll do better with a 6-millimeter lift. A majority of people with Morton's foot syndrome need at least 3.5 millimeters of correction, and almost half ultimately do better with 6 millimeters of correction.

These are very small dimensions and won't tilt your feet outward or force the inside of your feet upward to an unnaturally high level, like many orthotics do. They're simply meant to change how and when the foot senses the ground. As noted above, once that happens your neuromuscular system will do the rest.

If you think you need more lift, it would be best to confirm this with a practitioner who can help monitor your response to a higher amount of correction. Relatively few people need more substantial correction. But if you have chronic headaches, severe myofascial dysfunction, TMJ pain, pain in your arms or chest, or anxiety, you should see a trained practitioner who can more closely assess your posture and body mechanics.

After you've determined what correction you need, and after you have gotten new shoes, you can purchase a durable shoe insert. We recommend Posture Control Insoles, which you can purchase on our website (www.myopain.com) or at several other websites. We've seen hundreds of patients improve considerably after we've successfully fitted them with these insoles. This correction improves muscle function in many parts of the body and also reduces the sustained structural stress that can perpetuate trigger points and referred pain. Once you've corrected for Morton's foot syndrome, you'll need to follow the self-care guidelines for most of the muscles in this book.

Poor Footwear Choices

Another important perpetuating factor in low back and buttocks pain is poor footwear and wearing worn-out shoes. Many people simply do not replace their shoes once the sole is worn out. Shoes not only wear on the outside, where you can see it, but also within the sole, which may compress, changing the way you stand and walk. In addition, the human body just isn't cut out for wearing flip-flops on a regular basis. Not only do they make anyone's foot and leg muscles work too hard, they offer no support to the forefoot and are easily compressed. Anyone with Morton's foot syndrome should also be aware that flip-flops seriously exacerbate the problem. (By the way, if you have a hard time keeping your heels on top of flip-flops because they slide off to the inside, this is one of the clearest confirmations of Morton's foot syndrome.)

If any of the tests for Morton's foot syndrome indicate that you have foot problems, keep a close eye on all of your shoes for excessive wear. If the soles wear unevenly, replace or resole them as soon as possible. If you regularly wear flip-flops, it would be a good idea to replace them with a pair of well-designed sandals with a heel strap.

Short Upper Arms

If you have short upper arms, anytime you're seated in a standard office chair or something similar your elbows may not reach the armrests, so you have to tilt to one side or the other to allow at least one elbow to reach an armrest. This can lead to trigger points in the torso, low back, and neck, and in some cases may cause nerve compression and breathing problems. While this condition isn't very common, it can be a serious problem for those who have it.

Testing for Short Upper Arms

Shoulder pain, arm pain and dysfunction, mid and low back pain, and leaning to the side to reach an armrest are all indicators that you may have short upper arms. You'll need another person to help you do the following test to determine whether your upper arm bone (humerus) is short in relation to the rest of your body. Stand with your elbows bent and with your shoulders in a normal, relaxed position, making sure they aren't tight and elevated. Have the other person place their hands firmly against the sides of your waist and press onto the crest of your hip (the iliac crest). Note whether the tip of your elbow just meets the level of your iliac crest on each side. If your elbows are at least 3 inches higher than the crest of your hip when you stand in a completely relaxed position, you have short upper arms in relation to the length of your torso.

Correcting for Short Upper Arms

If your upper arms are short, some simple corrections can help you avoid adopting bad postural adjustments to compensate, often with painful consequences. First, try to use chairs with adjustable armrests. If that's not feasible, you can modify chairs by adding foam padding or pillows to raise the height of the armrests. When driving, you can use foam or pillows on the armrests. All of these adjustments will allow for relaxed, upright seated posture with support for your arms.

Problems Related to Poor Sleeping Position

If you sleep as much as most doctors recommend, you'll spend almost a third of your life in bed. So, as with breathing, it's worthwhile to carefully consider just how well you sleep and whether your sleeping position or sleep habits could be a perpetuating factor in your low back pain.

Poor Sleep Postures

If you're like many of our patients, you probably prefer one particular sleeping position, perhaps ever since you were a child. After interviewing thousands of patients over the past twenty-five years, we've found a high correlation of chronic pain with a face-down sleeping position, as shown in figure 17.3. Consider for a moment why sleeping on the abdomen can be so stressful. Imagine keeping your chest facing forward while you turn your head to look over your left shoulder at close to a 90-degree angle. Press your head into this position using your hand and see how long you can do it. This position involves actively contracting your neck muscles to allow your head to rotate and overstretching the other side of the neck. Now imagine lying in approximately this same position for the entire night. You can easily see how this can create a great deal of muscular dysfunction throughout the body. In addition to stressing the neck, this position chronically shortens one hip, which tends to contract the piriformis and the other gluteal

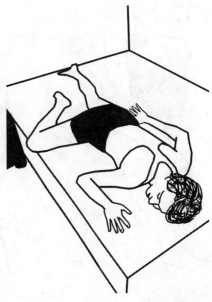

Figure 17.3

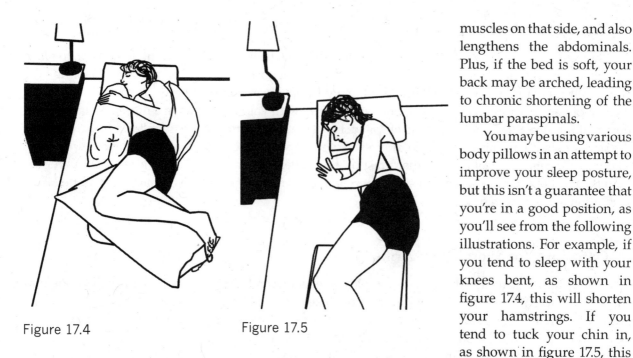

Figure 17.4

Figure 17.5

muscles on that side, and also lengthens the abdominals. Plus, if the bed is soft, your back may be arched, leading to chronic shortening of the lumbar paraspinals.

You may be using various body pillows in an attempt to improve your sleep posture, but this isn't a guarantee that you're in a good position, as you'll see from the following illustrations. For example, if you tend to sleep with your knees bent, as shown in figure 17.4, this will shorten your hamstrings. If you tend to tuck your chin in, as shown in figure 17.5, this thrusts your head forward and shortens the front of your neck. If you often sleep on your side with the upper leg dangling off the bed, as shown in figure 17.6, this overstretches your piriformis. Sleeping in the fetal position, as shown in figure 17.7, creates a host of problems: chronically shortened abdominals, iliopsoas, hamstrings, and pectoral muscles; chronically lengthened paraspinals; and head-forward posture which shortens the front of the neck. The asymmetrical position shown in figure 17.8 is also highly problematic, chronically shortening both hamstrings, the pectoral muscles, and the iliopsoas on one side, and chronically lengthening the piriformis and gluteal muscles on the other.

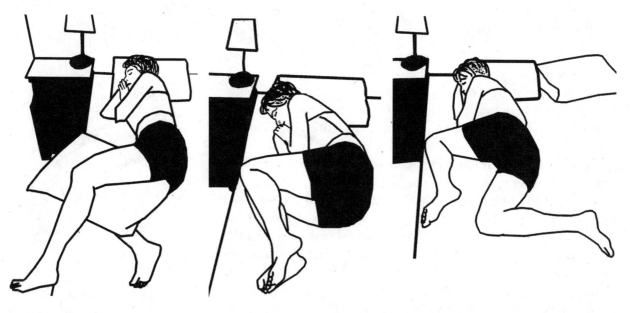

Figure 17.6

Figure 17.7

Figure 17.8

Good Sleep Postures

If any of those poor sleep positions look like you, you're probably wondering what you should do differently. Fortunately, relatively minor adjustments can make a big difference, so you should be able to find a modified position that works well for you. If you like to sleep on your side, you can significantly improve your position simply by using sufficient support under your neck and not bending either the hips or knees too much, as shown in figure 17.9. Also note how the support pillow between the legs extends from between the thighs all the way down to the feet. Another worthwhile adaptation is using a pillow alongside the front of your body, as shown in figure 17.10, to keep your chest and torso from collapsing inward. You can also place a pillow behind you, as shown in figure 17.11, as this allows you to rest your upper arm on the pillow behind you. This also helps open up and gently stretch the chest muscles, which tend to be chronically contracted for much of the day if you lean over a desk to work. Figure 17.12 shows a similar position with the addition of support under the hips to correct for a soft, sagging bed. However, if your mattress is too soft or worn out, you'd be well-advised to replace it as soon as possible. If the expense seems daunting, just remember how much of your life you spend in bed.

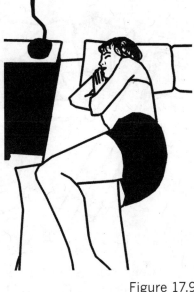

Figure 17.9

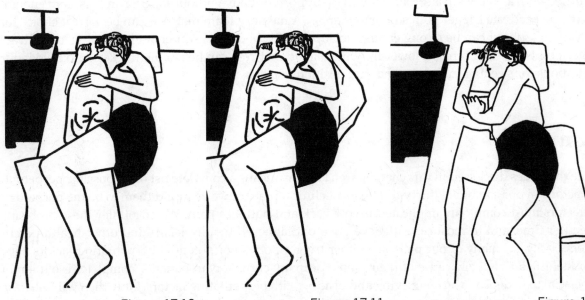

Figure 17.10   Figure 17.11   Figure 17.12

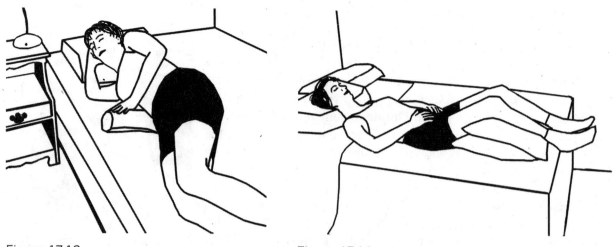

Figure 17.13   Figure 17.14

If your waist is much narrower than your hips, you may want to add some support under your waist, as shown in figure 17.13, so that your quadratus lumborum muscles aren't overcontracted on one side and overlengthened on the other. Sleeping on your back is a good option because it's easier to achieve a neutral position that doesn't overstress the body. Just be sure to use good support under your knees and neck, as shown in figure 17.14.

In general, it makes sense to get the very best bed you can afford. We've found that for most people, a firm bed with a pillow top is strong enough to support the body without sagging and also soft enough that it won't activate trigger points in tender areas. A memory foam mattress can be a great choice for the same reasons; it can be strong enough to support the body and soft enough that it won't activate trigger points in tender areas. However, while a good mattress can help a bit, the key is to follow our suggestions for sleeping in the most neutral position you can.

Summary

While the issues discussed in this chapter aren't by any means a complete list of all possible perpetuating factors, in our combined thirty-five years of clinical practice we've found them to be the perpetuating factors most commonly implicated in low back and buttocks pain. We encounter these problems time after time, and in most cases they've gone undiagnosed by physicians and other health practitioners. Sadly, for many of our patients neither trigger points nor potential perpetuating factors have been identified as a likely cause of their pain. For many chronic pain patients, complete resolution of myofascial pain depends on identifying and dealing with perpetuating factors. Only then will self-care fully resolve the problem. And if you're a therapist dealing with chronic pain, you can't do an effective job without understanding and learning to treat the conditions described in this chapter. We cannot overstress this point: Identifying and correcting for perpetuating factors often makes the difference between pain relief that's temporary at best and pain relief that's a complete and lasting resolution of the problem.

So whether you're a person suffering from chronic low back or buttocks pain or a therapist treating it, take time to consider all of the perpetuating factors discussed in this chapter. Use the tests we've outlined to determine which factors may apply, then be diligent about correcting any perpetuating factors you discover. This is the final challenge you must overcome if you are to be pain free.

To recap briefly, we hope this book has helped you understand the following important points:

1. Trigger points often play a central role in muscle pain.

2. Often, trigger points aren't located where the pain is felt.

3. There are predictable patterns of pain referral specific to trigger points in each muscle.

4. You can learn to apply effective and simple methods of treatment to your own dysfunctional muscles, using the appropriate tools as needed.

5. You may need to correct various perpetuating factors to achieve lasting pain relief.

For more information on where to obtain the tools recommended in this book, finding a trigger point therapist in your area, or training in myofascial trigger point treatment, visit our website (www.myopain.com). And of course, if you're in the Chicago area, you can also contact us to arrange for treatment in our clinic.

This book offers a different path to pain relief, one not dependent on drugs or surgery. Attaining lasting relief is hard work, especially when it entails a daily commitment and, in some cases, requires you to modify things as basic as the way you breathe, sit, eat, or sleep. Like so many things in life, you get back what you put into the process. We wish you the greatest success as you continue to use the self-care techniques you've learned in this book.

Appendix

Self-Care Quick Reference Guide and Summary of Tests for Muscle Dysfunction

For quick reference, the following illustrations show all the areas that might be treated for low back and buttocks pain. These illustrations combine all the figures in the muscle chapters offering guidance on where to do self-compression for each muscle. The larger X's represent the most likely places to find trigger points. However, because the entire length of a muscle can be dysfunctional, we recommend that you treat the entire muscle, as indicated by the small X's, applying more sustained compression to any areas that are firmer or more painful. And remember, before compression treatment it's a good idea to warm the area up, and after compression it's important to stretch the muscle (in a sequence with contraction and relaxation) and then do a few range of motion exercises for that muscle, which you'll find in chapter 16.

MYO Compression Protocol for Eliminating Low Back and Buttocks Pain Caused by Myofascial Trigger Points

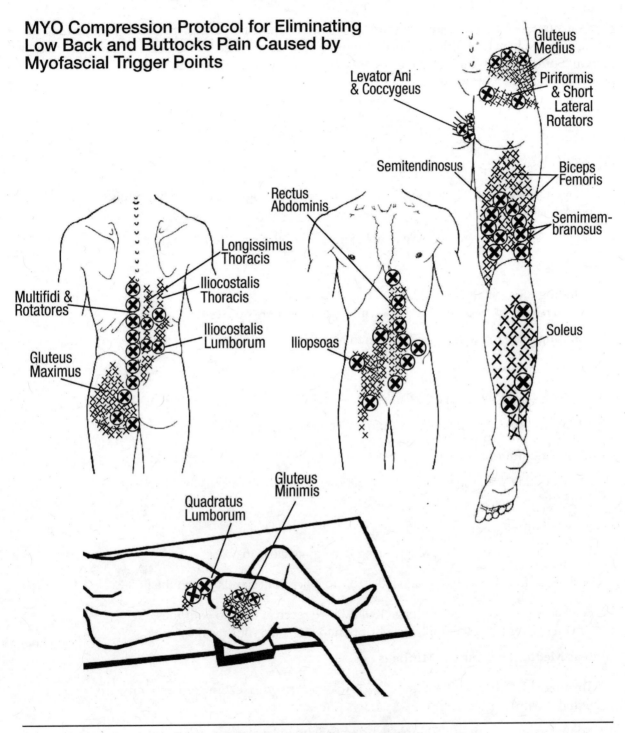

www.myopain.com

Summary of Tests for Muscle Dysfunction

Here's a summary of the range of motion tests that may indicate trigger points in various muscles. If you answer no to any question, read that muscle chapter and use the self-care techniques described therein. Some of the tests indicate a number of inches; in these cases we've indicated how to interpret your findings. Not passing a range of motion test doesn't always indicate trigger points; however, there's no harm in treating the muscle even if trigger points aren't present.

	Yes	No
Iliopsoas		
Seated chest to thighs (page 63): Able to bring chest to thighs with no pain in thighs or low back?	☐	☐
Straight leg raise (page 63): Able to hold legs up for 10 seconds without pain?	☐	☐
Paraspinals		
Standing toe touch (page 78): Able to touch floor with fingertips? (If you're over forty, see full test description to interpret your results.)	☐	☐
Standing torso rotation (page 79): Able to place both hands on the wall behind you?	☐	☐
Rectus Abdominis		
Abdominal roll-down (page 96): Able to roll downward slowly, to a count of 10?	☐	☐
Swing arm sit-up (page 96): Able to do the sit-up without pain?	☐	☐
Quadratus Lumborum		
Standing side bend (page 112): Able to get middle finger at least as low as top of kneecap?	☐	☐
Gluteus Maximus		
Knee to armpit (page 129): Able to bring knee quite close to chest?	☐	☐
Seated toe touch in a chair (page 130): Able to place your hands flat on the floor?	☐	☐
Seated toe touch on the floor (page 130): Able to reach at least to your toes? (If you're over forty, see full test description to interpret your results.)	☐	☐
Gluteus Medius and Gluteus Minimus		
Turning your feet in and out (page 137): Able to turn your feet inward and outward without pain?	☐	☐
Bonnet's sign test (page 137): Able to bring heel up to level of top of opposite knee without pain?	☐	☐
Pace abduction test (page 137): Able to push knees outward without pain?	☐	☐

	Yes	No
Standing leg swing out (page 137): Able to swing leg smoothly, without pain, difficulty, or cramping?	☐	☐
Knee crossing test (page 138): Able to easily cross upper knee completely over lower knee?	☐	☐

Piriformis

	Yes	No
Knee crossing test (page 138): Able to easily cross upper knee completely over lower knee?	☐	☐
Turning your feet in and out (page 137): Able to turn your feet inward and outward without pain?	☐	☐
Bonnet's sign test (page 137): Able to bring heel up to level of top of opposite knee without pain?	☐	☐
Pace abduction test (page 137): Able to push knees outward without pain?	☐	☐

Hamstrings

	Yes	No
Standing toe touch (page 78): Able to touch floor with fingertips? (If you're over forty, see full test description to interpret your results.)	☐	☐

Soleus

	Yes	No
Squat test (page 194): Able to bring buttocks fairly close to heels? (See the full test description to interpret your results.)	☐	☐
Standing toe touch (page 195): Able to touch floor with fingertips? (If you're over forty, see full test description to interpret your results.)	☐	☐
Single heel rise test (page 195): Able to raise up fully onto the ball of the foot?	☐	☐
Seated toe touch on the floor (page 130)	☐	☐

References

California HealthCare Foundation. 2008. Higher Rx spending drives U.S. health care costs above $2 trillion. *California Healthline*, January 8. www.californiahealthline.org/articles/2008/1/8/Higher-Rx-Spending-Drives-US-Health-Care-Costs-Above-2-Trillion.aspx?topicID=37. Accessed May 9, 2008.

Chaitow, L., D. Bradley, and C. Gilbert. 2002. *Multidisciplinary Approaches to Breathing Pattern Disorders.* London: Harcourt.

Fascia Research Congress. 2007. Terminology used in fascia research (prepared by Kim LeMoon). www.fasciacongress.org/2007/glossary.htm. Accessed June 17, 2009.

Ferguson, L. W., and R. D. Gerwin. 2004. *Clinical Mastery in the Treatment of Myofascial Pain.* Baltimore: Lippincott, Williams, and Wilkins.

Gerwin, R. D. 2005. A review of myofascial pain and fibromyalgia—Factors that promote their persistence. *Acupuncture in Medicine* 23(3):121–134.

Klein, M. J. 2006. Piriformis syndrome. www.emedicine.com/pmr/TOPIC106.HTM. Accessed June 6, 2008.

National Institute of Neurological Disorders. 2008. Low back pain fact sheet. www.ninds.nih.gov/disorders/backpain/detail_backpain.htm. Accessed May 9, 2008.

Plotnikoff, G. A., and J. M. Quigley. 2003. Prevalence of severe hypovitaminosis D in patients with persistent, nonspecific musculoskeletal pain. *Mayo Clinic Proceedings* 78(12):1463–1470.

Simons, D. G. 2002. Understanding effective treatments of myofascial trigger points. *Journal of Bodywork and Movement Therapy* 6(2):81–88.

Simons, D. G. 2004. Review of enigmatic MTrPs as a common cause of enigmatic musculoskeletal pain and dysfunction. *Journal of Electromyography and Kinesiology* 14(1):95–107.

Simons, David, MD. 2009. Information obtained from personal correspondence. December.

Simons, D. G., J. G. Travell, and L. S. Simons. 1999. *Myofascial Pain and Dysfunction: The Trigger Point Manual, Volume 1: Upper Half of Body.* 2nd ed. Baltimore: Lippincott Williams & Wilkins.

Taylor, Tim, MD and Anna Bittner, MD. 2009. Information on pages 233-234 from anecdotal and clinical evidence via personal correspondence. October-December.

Travell, J. G., and D. G. Simons. 1983. *Myofascial Pain and Dysfunction: The Trigger Point Manual. Volume 2: The Lower Extremities.* Baltimore: Lippincott Williams & Wilkins.

Travell, J. G., and D. G. Simons. 1992. *Myofascial Pain and Dysfunction: The Trigger Point Manual. Volume 2: The Lower Extremities.* Baltimore: Lippincott Williams & Wilkins.

Wang, J., B. O'Reilly, R. Venkataraman, V. Mysliwiec, and A. Mysliwiec. 2009. Efficacy of oral iron in patients with restless leg syndrome and low normal ferritin: A randomized double-blind placebo-controlled study. *Sleep Medicine.* 10 (9): 973-975.

Index

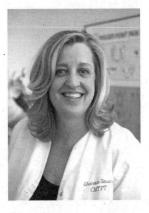

Sharon Sauer, CMTPT, LMT, is a myofascial trigger point therapist who has practiced in Chicago, IL, since 1986. She has successfully treated thousands of patients with chronic and acute soft tissue pain. Sauer has made significant contributions to the field of myofascial trigger point therapy, most notably, the incorporation of self-care training into treatment protocols for over sixty different kinds of myofascial pain and dysfunction. Sauer has been a featured speaker at the annual convention of the American Academy of Pain Management and has taught trigger point evaluation and elimination techniques to hundreds of doctors, osteopaths, dentists, chiropractors, physical therapists, massage therapists, and other health care practitioners.

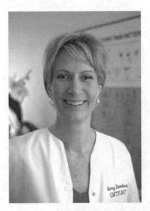

Mary Biancalana, MS, CMTPT, LMT, is a certified myofascial trigger point therapist in Chicago, IL, who has been treating chronic and acute soft tissue pain since 1999. She has been a personal trainer and fitness instructor since 1986. Biancalana has spoken extensively on complex myofascial pain syndromes and fibromyalgia, and has served as chairperson for the annual convention of the National Association of Myofascial Trigger Point Therapists. Biancalana has a particular interest in the detection and treatment of commonly overlooked perpetuating factors in chronic pain syndromes.

Foreword writer **Bernard E. Filner, MD**, is a practicing anesthesiologist and non-interventional pain medicine practitioner with more than forty years of experience. A leading expert on pain treatment, Filner has held faculty positions at the University of California at San Diego, the Columbia College of Physicians and Surgeons in New York, and the Department of Anesthesiology of George Washington University in Washington, DC. He now works in private practice, specializing in the treatment of myofascial pain and fibromyalgia.

For more information on the authors, consult www.myopain.com.

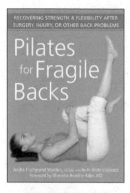
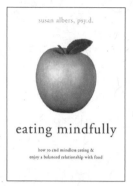
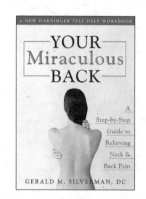
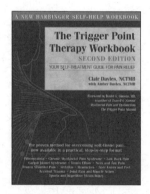
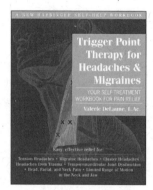
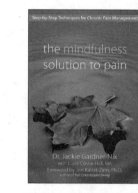
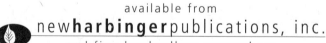